Wayne Matheson, PhD
Cornelius Van Dyk, BEd
Kenneth Millar, PhD

Performance Evaluation in the Human Services

Pre-publication
REVIEWS,
COMMENTARIES,
EVALUATIONS . . .

"**P**erformance Evaluation in the Human Services by Matheson, Van Dyk, and Millar is a refreshing 'real world' addition to the evaluation literature. The authors define the evaluation of employees as participatory and one which should be of equal benefit to the organization and employee. By setting a benchmark midpoint in the performance scale which 'specifies the organization's expected level of performance,' they have thereby set aside the remainder of the scale for professional growth and development. This unique approach allows individuals to 'charge ahead' in some years or 'rest up' in other years, while still meeting administrative performance standards.

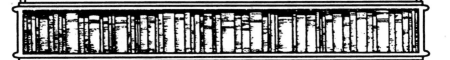

The authors develop an 'ideal' instrument that is multidimensional within two main areas. 'Core' dimensions are activities performed by everyone in the agency (ability to work effectively with colleagues) while 'àla carte' dimensions are job specific (establishment and maintenance of relationships with clients). This type of evaluation system successfully taps into the overall performance of the organization as well as individual performance. Finally, Matheson, Van Dyk, and Millar clearly define the process of evaluation and guide the evaluator and evaluated into a mutually beneficial outcome. This book bridges academia and the workplace and belongs on everyone's 'practical application' shelf."

Thomas R. Lawson, PhD
Director & Professor,
Raymond A. Kent School
of Social Work,
University of Louisville,
Louisville, Kentucky

" **T**he prevalent idea of this book is clearly stated by the words, 'The energy of the performance evaluation should be diverted towards a genuine responsiveness to the person being evaluated, and it should carry a message that there is something in it for everyone involved.' This philosophy is reinforced throughout.

As a supervisor it is very important to keep apprised of innovative methods to 'evaluate' staff, which benefits the staff person, the supervisor, and the agency. For too long we have done performance evaluations because we have to and not necessarily with the employee in mind. This book would be an extremely beneficial tool to the social services agencies."

Debra Shiell, MPA
Quality Assurance Coordinator,
Division of Children
and Family Services,
Arkansas Department
of Human Services

The Haworth Press, Inc.

Performance Evaluation in the Human Services

HAWORTH Social Administration
Simon Slavin, EdD, ACSW, Senior Editor

New, Recent, and Forthcoming Titles:

Social Administration, 2nd Edition by Simon Slavin
  Part I: *An Introduction to Human Services Management*
  Part II: *Managing Finances, Personnel and Information in Human Services*

Beyond Altruism: Social Welfare Policy in American Society by Willard C. Richan

Human Services Computing: Concepts and Applications by Dick Schoech

Lobbying for Social Change by Willard C. Richan

Research Utilization in the Social Services: Innovations for Practice and Administration edited by Anthony J. Grasso and Irwin Epstein

Social Work Ethics on the Line by Charles S. Levy

Community Organization and Social Administration: Advances, Trends, and Emerging Principles by Terry Mizrahi and John D. Morrison

Performance Evaluation in the Human Services by Wayne Matheson, Cornelius Van Dyk, and Kenneth Millar

Performance Evaluation in the Human Services

Wayne Matheson, PhD
Cornelius Van Dyk, BEd
Kenneth Millar, PhD

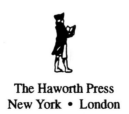

The Haworth Press
New York • London

The Haworth Press, Inc., 10 Alice Street, Binghamton, NY 13904-1580

Library of Congress Cataloging-in-Publication Data

Matheson, Wayne.
    Performance evaluation in the human services / Wayne Matheson, Cornelius Van Dyk, Kenneth I. Millar.
        p.   cm.
    Includes bibliographical references (p.   ) and index.
    ISBN 1-56024-379-1 (acid free paper).
    1. Human services personnel–Rating of. I. Van Dyk, Cornelius. II. Millar, Kenneth I. III. Title.
HV40.54.M37   1994
361.3′068′3–dc20   93-23223
                                                                                          CIP

CONTENTS

Preface   **ix**

Acknowledgements   **xiii**

Chapter 1. Performance Evaluation: An Overview   **1**

Introduction   1
Goals of Performance Appraisal   5
Common Performance Appraisal Mechanisms   6
The Ideal Performance Evaluation System   9

Chapter 2. Two Cases in Performance Evaluation   **13**

Ian Webster   13
Sally Abramson   17

**Chapter 3. The "Ideal" System for Human Service
Performance Evaluation**   **21**

Characteristics of the Ideal Process and Instrument
for Human Service Performance Evaluation   22

**Chapter 4. Constructing the Ideal Performance
Evaluation Instrument for a Human Service Agency**   **41**

Instrument Characteristics   41
Instrument Construction with Staff Participation   43
The Performance Evaluation Process   46

Chapter 5. The Performance Evaluation Instrument   **51**

Contents   51
Introduction   54
The Scale   54
The Dimensions   55
Time Boundaries   56
The Wording of the Dimensions   56
The Evaluation Process   56
Goal Setting Component of the Process   57

Performance Evaluation Instrument   59
Performance Evaluation Instrument Score Sheet   95
Comments   98

**Chapter 6. Implementing the Process/Using
the Instrument**   **99**

Introduction   99
"Ideal" Performance Evaluation   99
Keeping the Process Fresh   105

Chapter 7. The "Ideal" Performance System in Action   **107**

Applying the Synoptic and Focused Methods   108
The Synoptic Method   108
The Focused Method   110
The Systemic Method   111
The Synoptic and Focused Methods in Action   113
The Systemic Method in Action: A Clinical Team Review   120

**Chapter 8. The Ideal Performance Evaluation System:
Applications and Implications**   **123**

Staff Considerations in the Ideal System   123
Supervisor/Administrative Considerations in the Ideal
  System   126
Organizational Considerations in the Ideal System   129

References   **131**

Index   **137**

ABOUT THE AUTHORS

Wayne Matheson, PhD, C.Psych., is currently community services team manager, Child and Family Centre, Sudbury, Ontario.
Previously, he was visiting professor at the Centre for Research in
Human Development, Laurentian University, and Clinical Director
of South Cochrane Child and Youth Service, Timmins, Ontario.

Cornelius Van Dyk, BEd, is Executive Director, South Cochrane
Child and Youth Service. Mr. Van Dyk made a presentation to the
NASW on a Performance Evaluation Instrument. He serves on the
Board of Directors for the Ontario Prevention Clearinghouse.

Kenneth Millar, PhD, is Dean of the School of Social Work, Louisiana State, Baton Rouge. Formerly, he was Dean of the Faculty of
Professional Schools at Laurentian University. Dr. Millar has pub-
lished articles, presented at professional and academic conferences,
and conducted workshops in both the United States and Canada.

Preface

Much has been written recently of the need for the university to radically change its role vis-à-vis the community. Bok (1990) has spoken eloquently of the separation of academe from society and of the university's inability (or unwillingness) to address societal problems. Boyer (1990) has argued that the notion of scholarship must be expanded to include, among other things, the scholarship of application–how knowledge can be responsibly applied to consequential problems. Gilley (1990) notes that universities must become "others centered," a concept which involves far more than traditional ideas of service and includes the university reaching out to assist the community in defining how the university can be of service in solving its more difficult problems. He defines this as the "Interactive University: A university whose basic developmental strategy is to form an active and reciprocal partnership with the leadership (business, civic, and political) of its community or region, a partnership focused on the common goal of shaping a community that is strong and equitable, both economically and socially" (p. iii).

Schools of social work have not been immune to the criticisms leveled at the university for their failures in this regard. As the profession has sought credibility and legitimacy within academia, it has come to be seen by many as increasingly detached from the real world of practice, administration, and policy. In recent years, a number of people both inside and outside the university have tried to address this separation. A new (or renewed) spirit of partnership is developing between some members of the social work professorate and agency-based professionals, which is aimed at bringing the resources of the university to bear on specific issues and problems being encountered in the agency.

This text is the result of a successful university-agency collaboration. In the fall of 1988, two of the authors (Matheson and Van Dyk), both of whom were senior management personnel at the South Cochrane Child and Youth Service agency in Timmins, Ontario, sought assistance from the third author (Millar), who at the time was the Dean of the Faculty of Professional Schools and Professor of Social Work at Laurentian University, Sudbury, Ontario. The assistance requested was to cooperatively design, build, and implement a performance evaluation system for the agency.

The resulting four-year journey which has culminated in this book has not always been easy. Both parties to this enterprise have had to learn to speak each other's language, understand each other's motivations, goals, and aspirations, and appreciate each other's value system and philosophy. As the academic begins to work with the organization, he/she encounters a culture, a value system, a way of doing business, that is different from the one he/she is used to within the university. The university, grounded as it is in a tradition of research and scholarly writing, is often out-of-touch with the "real" world of work, even in an applied practice field such as social work.

The agency asks: "Will it work in our system?" and, "Is it consistent with our mission and our organizational structure and philosophy?" The university asks: "Does it advance knowledge?" "Is it defensible to the research community?" and (dare we say it?), "Is it publishable?" Yet, as Ann Weick (Marsh and Weick, 1992) reminds us, "Research questions seem to be as much driven by availability of funding, access to data, and tenure/promotion expectations as by a response to burning issues for which practitioners need help" (p. 140).

In addition, the scientific orientation instills a degree of conservatism in academics when it comes to problem solving–move cautiously, test, and evaluate. There is nothing inherently wrong with this approach. Indeed, it has a great deal of value. However, it is important to remember that the organization, in contrast, needs real answers to real problems–today, not tomorrow, next month, or next year.

The evaluation system implemented at South Cochrane Child and Youth Service had its beginning as a perceived problem within a service setting and a doctoral dissertation (Millar, 1988, 1990). The outcomes that resulted from our work together, first presented

as a paper at the 1989 NASW Annual Conference in San Francisco
and now more fully described in this text, are very different from
our initial effort. In the process both sides in the enterprise had to
relinquish entrenched positions, learn to accept and accommodate
opposite views, understand and appreciate different value stances
and philosophical orientations. The rewards in this endeavor were
well worth the effort.

Wayne Matheson
Sudbury, Ontario

Cornelius Van Dyk
Timmins, Ontario

Ken Millar
Baton Rouge, Louisiana

Acknowledgements

This book is the result of the contributions of many individuals who generously provided their assistance, support, and encouragement. In particular, a number of individuals associated with South Cochrane Child and Youth Services, Timmins, Ontario made this book possible. The authors would like to thank Mr. Ronald Bert, Executive Director; the members of the Board of Directors; and the staff, both past and present. A special word of gratitude is owed to Ms. Lucie Lamarche who typed many sections of the manuscript. Her excellent work, incredible patience, and diligence enabled us to meet all our deadlines.

Dr. Simon Slavin, the Editor of the Social Administration Series at The Haworth Press provided the authors with suggestions, advice, and support at many points during this project.

Last, but certainly not least, our heartfelt thanks and appreciation to our families, particularly our wives: Valerie, Rachelle, and Pat, for their constant support and the sacrifices they made to allow us the time to write.

Chapter 1

Performance Evaluation: An Overview

INTRODUCTION

The evaluation of employee performance is an annual occurrence in nearly all human service agencies, and the consequences of this evaluation for the individual being evaluated, the evaluator, and the organization can be quite profound. On the positive side, a well-conducted performance appraisal may:

- Increase the person's motivation to perform effectively;
- Increase the self-esteem of the person being evaluated;
- Allow new insights for the person or persons doing the appraisal;
- Result in more clarification and better definition of the job of the person being evaluated;
- Facilitate valuable communication among the individuals taking part;
- Promote a better understanding among participants, of themselves, and of the kind of development activities that are of value;
- Clarify organizational goals and facilitate their acceptance;
- Allow the organization to engage in human resource planning, test validation, and develop training programs.

On the other hand, a poorly conducted performance evaluation may:

- Cause individuals to quit as a result of the way they were treated;

- Create false and misleading data;
- Damage the self-esteem of the person being appraised and the person conducting the appraisal;
- Waste large amounts of time;
- Permanently damage the relationship among the individuals involved;
- Lower performance motivation;
- Waste money on forms, training, and a host of support activities;
- Lead to expensive lawsuits by those who feel unjustly evaluated. (Mohrman, Jr., Resnick-West, and Lawler III, 1989, pp. 3-5)

All too often, negative results are exactly what organizations get when they try to operate traditional appraisal systems. Frequently, the high hopes associated with a new performance evaluation system end up being destroyed by the reality of a system that produces more conflicts, problems, and resistance than positive results. In many organizations, performance appraisal systems simply become inoperative because of the problems and conflicts they generate. The challenge is to develop and implement a performance evaluation system that eliminates the many negative consequences and produces the important positive ones. Unfortunately, this is not an easy task.

Most people find the performance appraisal process a totally unrewarding, if not unpleasant, experience. Discomfort is often expressed by both supervisors and supervisees over the event (McGregor, 1972, Wiehe, 1980). Supervisors express anxiety at judging the performance of their supervisees, while the latter experience anxiety about being judged (Wiehe, 1980).

Supervisors frequently balk at the idea of performance appraisal because of: (1) an understandable dislike of criticizing a subordinate (and perhaps having to argue about it); (2) a lack of skill needed to handle the performance evaluation interview; and, (3) a mistrust of the validity of the appraisal instrument (McGregor, 1972). Cummings and Schwab (1973) add that supervisors may experience role conflict because of an inability to separate the judgmental/evaluative and educational/developmental components of performance evaluation. Supervisors also frequently lack an overall conceptual model of how appraisal contributes to other personnel functions such as recruitment, selection, placement, training, and utilization.

Rivas (1984), speaking expressly from a human services perspective, claims that evaluation is a troublesome process for supervisors because: (1) it specifically calls attention to the difference in status between supervisor and supervisee; (2) it reflects on the supervisor; (3) it can evoke strong negative feelings; and (4) it can be discouraging to workers.

Despite the inherent difficulties, evaluating performance is something that people do all the time. A great deal of informal evaluation takes place in organizations, just as it does in all sectors of people's lives. The performance of each individual in an organization is constantly being appraised by the individual, as well as by his or her supervisors, peers, and subordinates. Formal appraisal is an inevitable consequence of the way organizations are structured, and jobs are designed. The assignment of responsibility to particular individuals for the accomplishment of certain tasks makes the assessment of individual performance both possible and necessary: possible because it identifies the results for which the person is responsible; necessary, because complex, differentiated organizations need information about job performance in order to operate effectively.

But why is performance appraisal so difficult? On the surface, it appears simple: One individual observes another executing a task and reaches a judgement about how adequately that task has been performed. Such judging occurs regularly throughout all human endeavors, but the situation is substantially more complex in work organizations than it is in most situations where performance judgements are reached. Two characteristics make the appraisal of work performance unique: (1) frequently, the evaluator has reward power over the evaluatee; and, (2) the appraisal occurs in the context of an ongoing relationship.

The problem of performance evaluation in the field of human services is further compounded by the lack of "hard" objective measures. Performance often goes unobserved by human service system administrators because of the nature of the services provided and the confidential nature of the employee-client relationship. In addition, because the service technologies of the helping professions are not able to be specified as clearly as those of other professions or those of production, there remains an aura of mystery about what constitutes an effective and efficient service (Ferris, 1982; Rivas, 1984).

Performance appraisal in a service organization involves some of the most important aspects of people's sense of individuality and accomplishment since it deals with their competence and effectiveness. In addition, it is the point where the sometimes conflicting goals of organizations and individuals are addressed. It is also an activity that has important legal considerations and can lead to the courtroom. Most of all, perhaps, it is an interaction between two human beings, who often are nervous, tense, somewhat defensive, poorly prepared to discuss important issues, and full of their own misperceptions, biases, hopes, and values.

To use the words of Latham and Wexley, (1981, p. 2) ". . . performance appraisal systems are a lot like seat belts. Most people believe they are necessary, but they don't like to use them." As a result, evaluation systems are often used reluctantly to satisfy some formal organizational or legal requirement. However, employee evaluation remains an important management responsibility. Performance appraisal is crucial to the effective management of an organization's human resources, and the proper management of human resources is a critical variable affecting an organization's productivity. In addition, recent decisions by arbitration boards and the courts emphasize the importance for organizations to have well-documented objective records of employee performance relative to advancement, dismissal, or salary increases (Latham and Wexley, 1981; Wiehe, 1980).

In this book a substantially new way of approaching performance evaluation is proposed. However, before proceeding to a description of this model, a brief review of literature concerning the goals and mechanisms of performance appraisal is presented. An appreciation of this new approach will be enhanced by examining it in the context of traditional and commonly held views about this subject.

GOALS OF PERFORMANCE APPRAISAL

Performance appraisal systems are typically viewed as a contract between the organization and an employee explicitly specifying what is required of that individual. In this context, appraising performance is seen as necessary because it serves as an audit for the organization about the effectiveness of each employee. In effect, performance appraisal functions as a control system based on key job behaviors that serve as standards, which enable the manager to specify what the employee must start doing, continue doing, or stop doing. From this traditional viewpoint, performance appraisal fulfills two important functions: the counseling (motivation), and the development (training), of employees. It is on the basis of an employee's motivation and training that decisions are made regarding that employee's retention, promotion, demotion, transfer, or termination (Latham and Wexley, 1981).

There are also legal necessities for having a valid and reliable performance appraisal system in place. The courts have become increasingly concerned with the impact of an evaluation system on an employee's status within an organization.

For example, both Canada's Bill of Rights and Title VII of the 1964 Civil Rights Act in the United States affirm that it is against the law to affect an individual's status as an employee on the basis of race, color, religion, sex, or national origin. Although originally targeting unfair discrimination in the selection of employees, the courts and the Equal Employment Opportunity Commission in the U.S. have broadened their jurisdictional limits to include close scrutiny of any measurement tool ("test") or procedure that impacts on *any significant personnel decision*. Performance evaluations are viewed as "tests" which must be job-related and valid (Latham and Wexley, 1981). In both *Brito v. Zia Company* (1973) and *Wade v. Mississippi Cooperative Extension Service* (1974) the courts held that the rating systems in place were biased and not job-related. There must be (1) a relationship between the appraisal instrument and a job and (2) evidence that the appraisal instrument is a valid predictor of job performance.

The U.S. Civil Service Reform Act of 1978 puts even more responsibility on organizations to have valid and reliable performance appraisal systems in place. Section 430 of this act deals specifically with performance appraisal systems and states that performance standards must be based on *critical* elements of the job; that the manner in which these critical elements are established be recorded in writing; that the employee be advised of these critical requirements before rather than after the appraisal; and that most importantly, an employee appraisal must be based solely on an evaluation of his or her performance of these critical requirements.

COMMON PERFORMANCE APPRAISAL MECHANISMS

A variety of appraisal methods have been employed in an attempt to achieve these goals. Any evaluation system depends on the use of some kind of mechanism to form the basis of judging employee performance. The best appraisal mechanisms come closest to evaluating the behaviors that actually distinguish between successful and unsuccessful job performance. Any rating system used should be based on objective criteria. Although this may seem obvious to the reader, it is common for human service organizations to use arbitrary and subjective performance measures. The nature of many commonly used appraisal mechanisms makes their validity and reliability questionable and can easily lead to allegations of subjective evaluator bias.

Traditional Trait-Based Rating Scales

Most people have used (or have been subjected to), appraisal systems based on trait-based rating scales. Usually, a list of characteristics is presented and the assessor is asked to rate the employee on each quality listed. Ratings are usually on three-, four-, or five-point scales, from "excellent" to "poor" or "needs improvement," with gradations between.

The problem with these scales is that the characteristics listed are often vague and subjective. Evaluators are asked to rate employees in terms of their personal characteristics rather than in terms of specific skills or work-related behaviors. "Appraisal" of employees' initiative, enthusiasm, honesty, attitudes, or dependability is common.

Such ratings can be questioned on the basis of their fairness. Evaluator bias is a serious problem with such a rating instrument. Biases include a "halo effect," where the evaluator's total perception of the employee affects each separate rating, or a tendency among evaluators to: rate everyone as "average" (a central tendency effect); rate everyone "low" (a strictness effect); or, rate everyone "high" (a leniency effect).

Traditional rating scales are also limited in their practicality. If the purpose of evaluation is to improve performance, the mechanism used must point the way toward behavior that needs strengthening. If an employee receives low ratings on his or her personal characteristics, there is little that can be done to improve.

Ranking, Paired Comparison, and Forced Distribution Systems

In this method, each employee is compared with other employees in comparable positions in accordance with some criterion or criteria. The evaluator might rank employees from best to worst or compare each individual in turn with all others. There are a number of variations on the ranking method. In the paired comparison approach, the assessor is asked to first select the best and the worst employee along some criterion or criteria, then the second-best and second-worst, then the third, and so forth until all employees are ranked. The forced distribution variation specifies to the evaluator what percentage of the total number of employees can occupy a particular rank.

Ranking methods help make distinctions among employees when selections must be made for differential compensation or for promotion but they serve little other useful purpose. In fact, they have the potential for breeding distrust and cynicism about the performance appraisal system because employees frequently see little connection between their performance and how they are ranked. The tendency to promote unhealthy competition among employees is readily apparent and, like the trait-based scales, there is little guidance to the employee on how to take corrective action in order to improve performance.

Performance Tests

Tests of job-related skills are most often based on simulations, demonstrations, or work samples. Employees are asked to show they have the competencies related to effective job performance. This can work only if the system designers have validated the methods used and if the skills being tested can lend themselves to objective measurement. In human service work, the use of video or audiotapes of sessions with clients is an example of a performance test. Its use requires that the evaluators agree on what characteristics they want employees to demonstrate, and this can be a very difficult task. In addition, human service workers normally have a number of responsibilities beyond direct service delivery, so other appraisal instruments are required to supplement the skills test.

Critical Incident Techniques

Supervisors are sometimes asked to keep records of important incidents that demonstrate employees' strengths or weaknesses. Such documentation can provide data that can be used to give feedback to employees. The concreteness of recording events removes some of the bias that is found in trait-based rating scales but there remains a danger of subjectivity in the selection of which events to document. A halo effect can occur where supervisors seek positive or negative incidents that support their overall impressions of particular employees.

Behaviorally Anchored Rating Scales (BARS)

Critical incidents can be used as part of the process of developing behaviorally anchored rating scales. These scales are different from others in the way they are developed and in their focus on measurable employee behaviors rather than general traits. There are five major steps used in the development of BARS. First, people who are familiar with the job list specific incidents that would illustrate effective or ineffective performance. These incidents are then clustered into groups of performance dimensions. In order to provide for accuracy and objectivity, a second group of people, familiar with the work, matches incidents with dimensions–a process referred to as retranslation. The incidents are then scaled and a final instrument developed (Millar, 1990). The incidents that have been selected serve as "behavioral anchors" that translate important performance dimensions into concrete, behavioral terms.

The shortcoming of this approach is that many people must spend long hours developing the instrument. Once such an instrument has been developed, however, it saves time and effort by streamlining evaluation. This is because the tool can stand the test of time as well as the problems posed by different job descriptions and multiple programs. There is a potential for portability and universality in such an instrument and its capacity for involving employees in the process of evaluation is very high (Millar, Matheson, and Van Dyk, 1989).

THE IDEAL PERFORMANCE EVALUATION SYSTEM

The goals and mechanisms of performance evaluation described above have a legitimate place within any organization. Every organization must make informed and responsible decisions with respect to employee promotion, dismissal, retention, and so forth. All organizations must also have in place performance appraisal systems that are legally defensible in a court of law.

However, our concern is that all too often performance evaluation systems exist solely and exclusively to meet organizational needs and requirements. What frequently is forgotten is that there are two parties to the evaluation process and one of these, *the employee*, and his/her needs and aspirations, are accorded secondary status and importance. Unfortunately, employee entitlement and management responsiveness are characteristics found to be absent from virtually all performance appraisal systems.

We contend that the primary focus of the performance evaluation should be to:

- Promote professional growth and development;
- Involve staff with agency mandate and mission;
- Entitle staff to participation in the development and operation of their own evaluation system;

- Promote a sense of fairness about agency policies and procedures;
- Promote an organizational culture of equality and egalitarianism;
- Foster training and development opportunities; and,
- Promote creativity and a thirst for new knowledge in the field of endeavor.

We are certain that, if pressed, most social service agency executives and management personnel would assert that the performance evaluation system in place in their organization addresses each of these issues. Our experience, however, is that many workers in such agencies:

1. feel their professional growth needs get overlooked when in competition with organizational demands;
2. feel little sense of allegiance to the agency mandate and mission;
3. have a poor conceptual understanding of agency policies and procedures, particularly how these policies and procedures impact on their work;
4. mistrust, or at best, are wary of "management's" goals, practices, and "hidden agendas"; and,
5. have little incentive, or are given little encouragement to be creative, seek out new ways of doing things, experiment with new modes of service delivery, and so forth.

The "ideal" performance evaluation system is intended to redress these shortcomings. The next chapter presents two case examples of performance evaluation in action. The initial case demonstrates an example of a conventional appraisal, while the second describes our idea of how an evaluation should be conducted. The cases provide the background for the material which follows. Chapter 3 of the text introduces the reader to the characteristics of the "ideal" performance evaluation system. Chapter 4 discusses how the performance evaluation instrument and process are developed. In Chapter 5 a complete performance evaluation instrument and user's guide is presented, based on the material presented in the previous two chapters. Chapter 6 describes the implementation and use of the instrument and process, and Chapter 7 brings this material to life by presenting case material of the evaluation system in operation. Chapter 8 concludes with a discussion of our experience with this model and a discussion of its applicability in a variety of human service settings.

Chapter 2

Two Cases in Performance Evaluation

The previous chapter introduced the subject of performance evaluation, with particular focus on the potential negative and positive consequences of evaluation systems. This chapter discusses two case examples of performance evaluation in action. The picture of a weak evaluation system and process is presented in the case of Ian Webster. A faulty system and the equally poor manner in which the manager implements it is described and a sense of how this process leaves the employee feeling at its conclusion is conveyed.

In the example of Sally Abramson, a very different evaluation process is illustrated. In this case description, the reader will find all of the elements considered fundamental to an "ideal" performance evaluation system. The characteristics of the system are markedly different from the previous example, as well as the manner in which the system is implemented. Not surprisingly, the feelings of the employee at the conclusion of this evaluation are also dramatically different. In the cases of Ian Webster and Sally Abramson, the stage is set for the material encountered in Chapters 3, 4, and 5. In fact, it may be beneficial to return to this chapter after having read the next three.

IAN WEBSTER

Ian Webster arrived at work about fifteen minutes late, an unusual occurrence since he tended to be punctual to a fault and, in fact, normally was in his office at the Eastern Mental Health Center well before regular office hours. Today, however, unlike most days, Ian had not looked forward to coming to work and he had delayed his departure from home until the very last minute.

Today was Ian's anniversary date at the Mental Health Center and agency policy dictated that each employee be given an annual performance review at this time. Anticipation of this event caused Ian to look forward to this day with less than unbridled enthusiasm.

As he drove to work, Ian recalled last year's performance review. It was a rather unpleasant experience. His supervisor, Al Barton, informed Ian the day before the review that it would take place the next day. It was not only the late notice that upset Ian (he was forced to reschedule a number of appointments), but the manner in which it was done. Al stuck his head in Ian's office a half-hour before the end of the work day and said, "Oh, by the way, tomorrow's your anniversary date and we have to do your annual evaluation. Better review what we talked about last year and think about how the past year has gone. Get a copy of the evaluation instrument from the secretary and if you get the chance, take a look at it before our meeting."

That evening Ian spent a number of hours preparing for the following day's meeting. Just two years out of graduate school, he knew there were a number of things he did well but he was also aware that there were other areas of his performance that needed further development. Ian wanted to be open and honest about his perceived strengths and weaknesses but the instrument he had obtained from the secretary gave him a great deal of difficulty.

First, the form asked for ratings on vague and undefined characteristics such as his "adaptiveness," "flexibility," and "professional conduct." Since no guidelines were provided, Ian was immediately concerned that he and Al Barton might define these items in very different ways. Second, many of the areas of the instrument were not connected to his job, but instead seemed applicable to the staff who worked in the agency's residential child treatment center. Third, much of the instrument was written in language that Ian did not understand and which appeared to him to be nothing more than a "word salad." One question, for example, asked about his ". . . ability at negotiating the client-worker service interface . . . ." Finally, the scales were constructed in such a way that there was an implied admission of failure by acknowledging a weakness or the need for further growth and development in a particular area.

Despite these problems, Ian worked hard at considering the items on the instrument in a fair and comprehensive manner. Nagging at the back of his mind was the knowledge that it was also pay review time and he knew that this evaluation could, in large measure, determine his annual pay increase. He recalled asking himself as he prepared for his evaluation, "How can I be open and honest and focused on my professional development and yet not be judged in a way that does damage to my earning capacity and my career progression?" Ian never answered that question to his satisfaction.

Despite his reservations, Ian believed he had little to fear or worry about in his face-to-face meeting with his supervisor. He had always found Al Barton to be a reasonable and accommodating person and during their supervision sessions, when Ian had discussed problematic cases with him, Al had been supportive, encouraging, and helpful. However, what transpired proved to be very disturbing to Ian.

To start with, Al delayed the beginning of the meeting twice, telling Ian that he was dealing with ". . . some issues that simply can't wait . . . ." Ian remembered that when they finally did get together, Al gave the distinct impression that he would rather be somewhere else. During the course of their evaluation session, they were interrupted three times by phone calls and twice by people coming to Al's office door.

Ian was shocked to discover that his expectations for the ratings on many items were substantially different from Al Barton's actual scores. As he tried to discover the reason for this, he realized that the fear he experienced the previous evening, that he and his supervisor would define items in different ways, had, in fact, occurred. For example, a particular incident which Ian felt had demonstrated his use of professional principles and the appropriate use of professional authority was considered by Al to show ". . . lack of flexibility . . . ." The items that Ian had wryly described as "a word salad" proved even more problematic in this regard.

The items that Ian thought had nothing to do with his job also caused trouble in the face-to-face meeting. Ian had thought that many of these items would be left blank or marked "NA" for "Non-Applicable" and others would be modified or changed to better reflect his job. Mr. Barton had done neither of these things. Rather, he had evaluated Ian on each item as it was written in the instrument. When Ian protested, Al explained that every item needed to be completed ". . . in order to get a cumulative score . . . ."

Given this situation, it is not surprising what transpired. The meeting degenerated into one where both parties actively defended and advocated for their own positions. While there was some give-and-take and an attempt to find compromise, little was accomplished. Ian felt pressured during the entire session to accept Al's evaluation.

There were other elements of the evaluation that disturbed Ian. On occasion, and in order to defend his position, Al made reference to aspects of Ian's performance that had occurred *prior to the last evaluation*. Later, Ian recalled how decidedly unfair he considered this tactic. That year had been his probationary period, his first year out of graduate school. Also, Ian believed that he and Al had "signed off" on that year and that this evaluation was to be specifically for the past twelve months.

The conclusion of the session was equally unsettling. Despite having spent a good deal of time on Ian's past and present performance, no mention was made of the future. The meeting ended without any identification of goals or objectives to be aimed for or reached in the coming year.

Ian was deeply upset about the evaluation process for weeks after its occurrence. He felt that some of his fundamental rights had been violated, and he was left with little sense of accomplishment for the past year and with even less sense of direction for the coming year. Furthermore, he was concerned about how the evaluation would impact his salary increase and his subsequent chances for promotion within the agency. Finally, he worried about how the evaluation process would affect his ongoing relationship with Al Barton.

Some of his worries proved to be unwarranted. He was relieved (in a way) when the Board of Directors approved an across-the-board pay increase rather than one based on merit. He found that Al continued to be helpful and supportive in his day-to-day supervision. Nevertheless, the feeling of disappointment persisted and he found himself becoming increasingly cynical about the evaluation process. He also started to protect himself, making prodigious notes of his activities and, more importantly, his conversations with Al and other senior staff. To his surprise and dismay, he discovered that his co-workers shared his cynicism.

SALLY ABRAMSON

Sally Abramson was in high spirits as she prepared to meet her husband for lunch. That morning she had completed her annual evaluation with her supervisor, Marge Peters, and she was looking forward to discussing its outcome with her husband. She had reason to feel pleased. The evaluation process, as it always was at her agency, had been a positive experience. She and Ms. Peters had not agreed on all items, but their differences had been amicable and mutually respected. More importantly, the meeting had concluded (as it had the previous year) with a clear delineation of expectations and objectives for the twelve-month period ahead.

As she walked to lunch, Sally thought to herself that her agency conducted performance evaluation "the right way." First, the instrument used in her evaluation had been developed through a series of meetings between management and staff. In hindsight Sally thought that this process, though time-consuming and at times frustrating, had been well worth the trouble. She believed the instrument was specifically related to her job and, just as important, was written in job-related language that she and the other workers could all understand and approve.

Sally had not heard of many organizations that had an evaluation instrument quite like the one in place at her agency. First, the staff and management had agreed on a number of job dimensions that were "generic" to all staff in the organization. In other words, despite the position an individual held on the organizational ladder or the nature of his/her specific job, this generic "element" was to be evaluated. "Establishment and Maintenance of Purposeful Relationships with Colleagues" was one such element. The Executive Director liked to refer to these as "Core" dimensions.

Then, recognizing that in a multi-faceted agency such as theirs not everyone performs the same functions, each job group had developed a set of specific components relating to their tasks and duties. For example, one of Sally's was called "Problem Identification and Assessment." On the other hand, Sally's supervisor, Marge

Peters, did not see clients and hence did not have this job aspect included in her evaluation package. In contrast, her evaluation included "Management of Human Resources." Around the agency, these items were lightheartedly referred to as the "À La Carte" dimensions.

There were other aspects of the evaluation instrument that Sally liked. After the components were identified and defined, each of them was "grounded" in a series of behavioral statements that reflected varying degrees of competence and proficiency. In retrospect, Sally realized that this had perhaps been the toughest job of all in the instrument construction.

A nice feature of the resulting scale was that it clearly demarcated the administrative requirements included in each dimension from those of professional growth and self-development. The midpoint of each dimension was referred to as the "benchmark" and reflected the minimum behavior expected by the agency in that work component. Below this point were descriptions of behaviors that were of concern to the organization. Above the "benchmark" were examples of behaviors associated with professional growth and development.

The entire evaluation instrument was bound in a manual. It included a guide that gave helpful information on how to use it. The manual also listed and defined each dimension and presented each complete scale. Sally had been part of the establishment of the evaluation system and had received her copy of the manual upon its completion. Also, the manual was now given to each new employee as part of their orientation, accompanied by extensive discussion between the employee and his/her supervisor about its use.

Sally also felt good about the process of the evaluation. A month ago, Ms. Peters had sent her a memo, reminding her that her annual evaluation was approaching and that she should complete the evaluation instrument independently. Marge Peters had also scheduled a meeting for two weeks hence, to be used for discussion of their scores. This meeting had gone well. After Sally had shared her scores, Ms. Peters had focused on the three dimensions where their scores differed by more than one point on the scale. This was followed by a discussion of the other dimensions. Neither of them felt any particular pressure to change their ratings and the mood of the meeting was positive and upbeat. Sally particularly appreciated the way her supervisor had dedicated this time to her, keeping the session free from distractions and interruptions.

The meeting had concluded with a brief discussion of goals and objectives for the coming year and they had set another meeting to discuss this aspect more fully. This was the meeting that had occurred this morning. Based on the evaluation, the two women identified a set of goals for Sally to accomplish over the next twelve months. Some of these dealt with Sally's concern that she was at the "benchmark" on two scales and she wanted to concentrate on her professional growth and development. On "Organization of Work and Time Management," Ms. Peters had rated Sally below the "benchmark" and they then identified means of addressing this issue over the coming year. During the meeting, Sally had mentioned one aspect of her job that she felt had changed and it was agreed that the dimension covering this would be discussed and possibly modified or changed at the next meeting of the job group. At the conclusion of the meeting, Sally and Ms. Peters had "signed off" on the instrument.

As Sally was to later tell her husband over lunch, she felt enthusiastic about the entire process. She believed she had played a central role in her evaluation; she had identified areas in which to grow and develop over the next year, and had acknowledged one area of weakness and determined the action necessary to improve it. Most of all, she felt valued and empowered and good about herself and the job she does.

Chapter 3

The "Ideal" System
for Human Service
Performance Evaluation

A good performance evaluation system should meet three criteria: it should be valid; it should be reliable; and it should be practical. Validity refers to the degree to which an instrument is measuring what it is supposed to measure. Reliability involves the extent to which a measurement gives consistent numerical descriptions of individuals from one time to another or from one evaluation to another. Practicality refers both to the instrument's acceptability to management and staff, and its accessibility, ease of administration and interpretation, and time required for completion (Baker and Holmgren, 1982; Millar, 1990; Smith, 1976; Wexley and Yukl, 1977).

This chapter delineates and then describes a set of characteristics of performance evaluation which, when present, accomplish a number of objectives. First, they ensure that the performance evaluation process and instrument satisfy the validity, reliability, and practicality requirements described above. Equally important, they provide assurance that the evaluation system will be seen as fair and appropriate by its users. The characteristics of the "ideal" performance evaluation system also guarantee a sense of responsibility and ownership that can reduce and even eliminate the feelings of anxiety, suspicion, and insecurity that frequently accompany performance evaluation.

CHARACTERISTICS OF THE IDEAL PROCESS AND INSTRUMENT FOR HUMAN SERVICE PERFORMANCE EVALUATION

1. Is positive and non-punitive in intention and design.
2. Emphasizes administrative requirements as well as self-development and professional growth on each dimension.
3. Includes both generic (CORE) and job-specific (À LA CARTE) dimensions.
4. Uses a benchmark to indicate the level of agency expectation.
5. Is not associated with pay or increments.
6. Uses simple, commonly understood language.
7. Is built with staff participation.
8. Describes and is anchored in real events.
9. Is time-framed and repetitive.
10. Has a user's guide.
11. Is future-oriented in operation.
12. Is fast and efficient.
13. Has an independent component completed in advance.
14. Is non-adversarial and allows for disagreement.
15. Is responsive to both development and diminution in ability over time.
16. Is available immediately upon employment as well as throughout an individual's employment.
17. Has high content validity.
18. Generates a sense of fairness.
19. Is a personalized experience.
20. Has a goal orientation step as a part of closure.
21. One instrument fits all staff.
22. Can grow and change with the agency.
23. Is comprised of both semantic and numerical components.

1. Is Positive and Non-Punitive in Intention and Design

Lombardi (1988) understates the issue when he declares that "the common problem with performance appraisal is that there is not a positive purpose to the whole exercise" (p. 147). It often appears that the main intention of performance evaluation is to use the results solely to manage the human resources of the agency in the promotion of the economic and administrative efficiency of the overall operation (Levine, 1986; Rendero, 1980). As a result, the system is frequently seen as nothing more than a control device which is inherently punitive.

Performance evaluation must communicate a positive message. Unfortunately, all too frequently it tends toward a critical appraisal rather than a supportive, conjoint evaluation. Indeed, performance appraisal can be so negatively perceived that "unless handled with consummate skill and delicacy, constitutes something dangerously close to a violation of the integrity of the personality" (McGregor, 1972, p. 134). To present a positive image, the evaluation must be seen as being driven by an overriding concern for the person being evaluated. A more predictable pattern, regrettably, is that appraisal is done *for* organizations and *to* people and the average employee takes six months to recover from the impact (Peters, 1985).

A critical point, then, is to orient the process and the instrument toward a positive intention and a constructive process. The goal is to reduce, wherever possible, the negativism frequently associated with the performance evaluation concept and to drive toward an optimistic outcome. Simply stated, this outcome is to help employees in ways they would like to be helped as well as in ways others (peers, supervisors, etc.) would like to see them improve. Both goals are relevant but the latter one should not be the overriding thrust of the process. The energy of the performance evaluation should be directed toward a genuine responsiveness to the person being evaluated and it should carry a message that there is something in it for everyone involved. After all "the conditions under which this judgement of quality is made, and the safeguards for the employee, are among the most important questions of social justice in industrialized societies" (Jacques, 1976, p. 55). Each of the characteristics which follow is premised on the initial assumption that the performance evaluation system is positive and non-punitive in design.

One final point should be made before proceeding further. The discerning reader will have realized by now that we are talking about far more than the performance evaluation system here. The method by which organizations evaluate their employees is a statement about their entire philosophy and culture. Organizations meta-communicate about their management style in their policies, programs, and protocols. The performance appraisal process, and its associated instrument, makes a statement–a metacommunication–about the attitude and posture of the agency toward its employees. The positive, non-punitive approach to performance evaluation is a fundamental statement about what the organization considers important and is a reflection of the way it carries out its business with external constituents, including its consumers.

2. Emphasizes Administrative Requirements as Well as Self-Development and Professional Growth

Keeping a performance evaluation system positive and non-punitive is a challenging task if one tries to direct the instrument and process toward both administrative concerns and self-development and professional growth. Combining judgmental and developmental dimensions on the same instrument is a difficult step (Cedarblom, 1982), since it is widely held that one of the problems with performance evaluation is that its administrative and developmental objectives are contradictory (Brumback, 1988). We propose the way to manage this problem is by using a "benchmark" (see Characteristic 4). In our system, the first few steps on any performance dimension scale deal with administrative concerns, and the "benchmark" specifies the organization's expected level of performance and the ceiling of administrative expectation. The remainder of the steps on the scale, beyond the benchmark, are oriented specifically toward professional growth and development. Chapter 4 speaks in more detail about the construction of this form of performance dimension scale and Chapter 5 gives illustrations of how they appear.

This approach to building dimensions with benchmarks for administrative expectations is far better than the more typical performance evaluation scaling which provides a ceiling of "perfection." Brumback (1988) remarks that ". . . placing unreasonably high expectations upon individuals can create a breeding ground for discontent, hypertension, protest, and cutting corners, including ethical and legal ones. True leadership, in our opinion, allows each individual to decide whether to strive beyond reasonable expectations and makes clear the individual will also be held accountable for his or her manner of striving. An organization can be more sure that its expectations are reasonable by keeping them job-related. That is, consistent with each individual's duties and responsibilities" (p. 391).

The more traditional approach invariably leads to one of two outcomes. Either "grade inflation" occurs as everyone, or nearly everyone, is ranked at or near the top of the scale (a leniency effect) or, the scale is seen as punitive and defeatist, particularly by younger or less-experienced staff, because it sets unrealistic and unattainable expectations of performance. In either case, the notion of professional growth and development is defeated by the performance evaluation instrument.

Lombardi (1988) has concluded that "virtually every attrition study done in the human resources field has found that a major reason for an employee leaving one firm for another is the well-formed impression that the former employer was uninterested in the employee's long-term development" (p. 157). The effort here, then, is to try to respond to this concern by building the two components of administrative expectation and developmental issues together on each and every dimension of the scale. The two components are together but are separated by the "benchmark" or administrative ceiling where the employee can satisfy organizational demands and still have room to move upward on the professional development range of the scale.

3. Includes Both Job-Specific Criteria and Generic Dimensions

A critical feature of any performance evaluation process is that the person should be evaluated against his or her actual job description, and that the criteria for evaluation are both objective and familiar to the participants (Latham and Wexley, 1981; MacIntosh, 1988). Invariably, of course, more than what is stated in the job description is expected of any employee (Lombardi, 1988). For example, every human service organization expects its employees to represent the agency appropriately and to behave with professional integrity in their working roles. These responsibilities are not always articulated within the job description but nevertheless should be a part of any evaluation process. (Harkness and Mulinski, 1988; Spano, 1981).

To be comprehensive, a performance evaluation needs to address both aspects of a job–those that are specifically and clearly outlined in the job description and those that are more generic or "core" for any individual working in a human service agency. Each employee should be made aware of these generic aspects of performance expectation as well as those that are more formally outlined in the job description.

This notion of discriminating between generic aspects of work and more specific job description components may appear unclear. Here is an example. Few would argue that a job dimension such as "Establishing Relationships with Colleagues" is a universal expectation for individuals in human service work. It is a dimension that has generic relevance and importance. It applies to everyone, irrespective of one's particular job station. However, consider a dimension entitled "Designing an Intervention Plan." Not everyone who works within a human service agency is charged with the task of "designing an intervention plan." This dimension speaks to a particular job group within a service system–one that deals directly with clients. Designing intervention plans is not a generic expectation. This dimension is not applicable to everyone in the system, and certainly not in the way that "establishing relationships with colleagues" is. One is generic and one is job specific. We have labeled generic job expectations "CORE" dimensions and for reasons that will become obvious, those that are specific to a job description we have called "À LA CARTE" dimensions.

The instrument, then, should be built to reflect both aspects of a job–those dimensions which address the actual job description, and those which address the more generic components of professional practice. This combination of elements makes the performance evaluation process and instrument more comprehensive. This combination of elements receives support from Kagle (1979), who argues that knowledge of generic evaluation principles can strengthen standards, in addition to other evaluative criteria that can be developed by agencies for particular programs.

We recommend the procedure whereby all employees are evaluated on an agreed-upon set of generic dimensions (CORE) while more discriminating job description dimensions (À LA CARTE) are selected by individuals or job groups. In this way, the instrument is very flexible and yet all-embracing and universal. The À LA CARTE job description dimensions can reflect all potential job roles and can continue to be added, amended, or deleted as the agency changes, while the CORE dimensions remain basically stable across time.

Subsequent chapters describe more fully the differences between CORE and À LA CARTE dimensions and how they are selectively combined to create a performance evaluation instrument that is unique for each employee.

4. Uses a Benchmark Level of Agency Expectation

The separation of agency expectations and professional development on each and every evaluation dimension is a fundamental strength of the form of performance evaluation being proposed. Both components are essential to the evaluation protocol but are rarely found together in one instrument, let alone on each dimension of the instrument. Often, organizational expectations are considered paramount and the issue of professional growth is reduced or even eliminated from the evaluation.

In the ideal instrument, the two components appear together on every dimension of the scale. It becomes, as described above (see Characteristic 2), a two-dimensional evaluation instrument. The scale is divided by the use of a benchmark, a feature that was mentioned previously and now described more fully.

The benchmark specifies the organization's expected level of performance on a particular dimension of the scale. Usually, the benchmark is point #4 on a 7-point scale or, in other words, the mid-point on the scale. Each dimension, then, has a "ceiling" of administrative expectation. The remaining points on the scale (five through seven), are concerned with aspects of professional growth and development. In effect, they deal with an employee's individual goals rather than organizational goals and expectations.

A contentious issue in performance evaluation is addressed through this benchmark distinction between agency expectation and professional growth and development. This is the distinction between the judge/evaluator role and the helper/counselor role. (Sashkin, 1981). The benchmark concept eliminates this antagonism and allows a presentation of both perspectives. The agency has an opportunity to address limitations and weaknesses in expected levels of performance, but those employees who have already reached the agency expectation (the benchmark) can focus on areas of professional growth and development.

The concept of the benchmark may be difficult to understand in the abstract. This characteristic is described more fully in the next chapter and in Chapter 5 where a complete evaluation instrument is presented. Chapter 5 also shows concrete examples of how the benchmark combines organizational expectations and professional development and growth on the same scale.

5. Is Not Associated with Pay or Increments

The initial purpose of performance evaluation is to measure the ability of staff to meet the administrative standards of performance. When this has been determined, the next concern is professional growth and improved performance over time. The performance evaluation process must be clearly seen by all players as disconnected from any reimbursement and not directly related to pay or financial value to the agency. We have already emphasized that the performance evaluation process must be seen as positive and non-punitive. For this reason, it is important that it should not be tied to any formal relationship with annual increments, bonuses, or financial incentives. (Patten, 1976; Patz, 1975; Rock, 1972; Wiehe, 1980). These two aspects of work–performance evaluation and re-muneration–should be separated. They should occur in different contexts and at different times in the working life of the employee (McGregor, 1972). To tie the two issues together is to connect performance evaluation with a management decision around the monetary value of the staff member. To associate the performance evaluation with a financial consequence also distracts from the true intent of performance evaluation–encouraging competence, objective appraisal of skill, and the planning of goals and personal development. Frequently the employee will be unwilling to be self-critical if reimbursement issues are contingent upon a successful evaluation. The whole process can become stilted and lacking in genuineness and honesty (Lombardi, 1988). The issue of pay, increments, and bonuses should be dealt with in the policy and procedures manual as a separate mechanism.

6. Uses Simple, Commonly Understood Language

The language of the evaluation instrument must be free of jargon, buzzwords, and generalizations. It must be germane to the participants and their job functions. Here are a few examples of the language that can appear in performance evaluation instruments:

> "Worker can successfully integrate the complementary components of service interface"; or,

> "Operates with an understanding of conjoint, client-service provider influence in intervention processes . . . ."

Clearly, such performance descriptors have little meaning or relevance and do little more than invite cynical comments from employees.

Additionally, the instrument must be cleansed of words that are so comprehensive and all-encompassing that they lack any specificity. Words that are difficult to define and to measure such as "frequently," "continually," "occasionally," "absolutely," and "persistently" come to mind.

These "traps" of language should be avoided as much as possible. They rob the instrument of its credibility, appropriateness, and usefulness. The performance evaluation instrument is of little merit if the language of the tool is not understood by the target group.

One way to accomplish this is to involve the employee group in the development of the performance evaluation instrument. This will help ensure that the instrument is written in job-relevant language that has meaning to the group who will eventually be evaluated by it.

7. Is Built with Staff Participation

Involving employees in the development of the evaluation instrument has rewards other than ensuring that it has job-relevant language that is easily understood. A performance evaluation process or instrument needs to be concerned about staff empowerment. Spano (1981) declares that staff should "have participation in developing and shaping all aspects . . ." (p. 4). The loyalty and commitment of staff to any evaluation process is virtually impossible without their input and involvement at every step–from conception to finished product.

Most performance evaluation tools are not built in this fashion. Often they are purchased or borrowed and then altered or modified to accommodate the host organization. Lacking employee input, they rely on management's knowledge and appreciation of the tasks performed in any job.

The input of management should not be undervalued but, as with Pottinger and Goldsmith (1979), we take the position that this "expert opinion" approach is the least valid method of competency evaluation. Furthermore, the "experts" may be involved in administration or training more than in the actual practice of the profession and tend to emphasize attitudes that in practice are relatively unimportant (Kane, 1982).

In reviewing the performance appraisal literature Evans and McShane (1988) report that with few exceptions, employees have more positive attitudes toward appraisal when they are given the opportunity to participate. Furthermore, the contribution through staff participation is considered a major element in successful appraisal systems, particularly when combined with problem solving and mutual goal setting (Nemeroff and Wexley, 1979; Wexley, Singh, and Yukl, 1973).

8. Describes and Is Anchored in Real Events

The performance evaluation instrument should confine its content to those dimensions that actually occur in the job. This may appear to be stating the obvious but it is remarkable how frequently items appear in an evaluation instrument that have absolutely nothing to do with a particular job. As Baker and Holmgren (1982) remind us, the process must be seen to be measuring the "right" things. To repeat what we have already said about staff involvement, these "right" things are most often best obtained from employees familiar with the job and, as a result, can generate context-specific material that can be used in the building of the instrument (Atkin and Conlon, 1978; Ferris, 1982).

Employee involvement is accomplished by promoting the value of staff experience, training, and knowledge, and demonstrating how these qualities can be utilized in the design of the evaluation process and the construction of the instrument. Lombardi (1988) identifies the situational relevance of evaluation items as one of the ten traits of a fair and effective review.

A further advantage of a performance evaluation instrument and system which is grounded in specific job-related behavioral content is that it is more easily defensible in courts of law. In this book we are emphasizing the positive and empowering aspects of performance evaluation. Nevertheless we must never lose sight of the fact that an evaluation may be challenged legally.

9. Is Time-Framed and Repetitive

The performance evaluation system must be communicated to each employee as a process framed in time. Each employee should be evaluated annually and at a time which he/she finds easy to remember. Most organizations will find it easiest to use the anniversary date of initial employment for subsequent evaluations. Frequently, new employees are reviewed after six months of probationary employment and then at subsequent anniversary dates.

Whatever the method for determining review dates, it is most important that the evaluation encompasses only the time period between reviews. It is also important that the performance evaluation not focus on more recent events, or isolated incidents, at the expense of the overall "pattern" of performance throughout the total period of the review.

When a performance evaluation instrument is repeatedly used across evaluations, the instrument should be capable of reflecting patterns of improvement and change. The repetition of the same evaluation process is a key to its success (Landy, Barnes, and Murphy, 1978). Unfortunately, many employees are never evaluated and, when they are, it is not repeated across their work experience. Frequently, evaluation instruments are changed between reviews. As a consequence of both these occurrences, change and development are not measured.

10. Has a User's Guide

An ideal performance evaluation instrument includes a user's guide with the instrument. The guide takes all parties to the evaluation through the process and the instrument. It outlines the scales and how they are designed. It describes the dimensions and tells the reader what the dimensions are attempting to measure. The guide removes vagueness and confusion from the instrument and provides an opportunity to make certain there is a shared understanding about the evaluation. Additionally, and sometimes more importantly, the guide tells the user what not to do, and what not to be concerned about.

11. Is Future-Oriented in Operation

Performance evaluation focuses primarily on the past: what the employee has done since the last review; and the present: the employee's current level of performance. Another consideration should address using this present and past information to deliver a message about future expectations. Reviewing the status of performance evaluation, Levinson (1979) suggests that one of the main problems is that it remains too long in the past. The consideration of future goals and objectives and what might be required (training, education, "re-tooling," etc.) to reach these goals should become a featured component of the evaluation system.

By including a future component to the evaluation process, management communicates that it is interested in the long-term professional development of employees. This is important for a number of reasons. Staff retention is one. Concern about employee retention is of particular importance in human service agencies where professionals are costly to recruit and to train. Most have university training and many have graduate-level degrees which provides them with considerable mobility. They can be easily driven away because of appraisal systems which they perceive as being punitive and which pay little attention to their future professional development.

A future-oriented evaluation system also allows an organization to more accurately and effectively plan educational, training, and other developmental activities for employees. Frequently, organizations invest inordinate amounts of time and money on activities that *management* thinks important for its staff. Managers are then surprised, and frequently, bitter, cynical, and even angry, when employees express and/or demonstrate little enthusiasm for these programs. The problem, of course, is that these activities often have little relevance to what employees believe are their development needs. A future-orientation ensures that staff development efforts will be accepted by staff and will be cost-effective.

A future-focus also allows for career planning with employees and facilitates better decision making, and more acceptance of internal promotions and transfers.

12. Is Fast and Efficient

No part of the performance evaluation process should require extraordinary lengths of time to complete. No part of the process– from the personal appraisal completed individually, to the joint evaluation interview, to sign-off, should require more than one hour of time for each session. A total of three hours should be all that is required to complete the entire evaluation process. Sometimes, the paperwork and technical assistance required by the appraisal system places an unreasonable workload on managers (Sashkin, 1981). This can be a deterrent to proceeding with the evaluation and gives the whole function a burdensome tone. Failing to streamline the process can even interfere with agency effectiveness (Wexley and Yukl, 1977). Performance evaluation should not be burdensome, either to employee or manager and it can easily become so if the time requirements become overwhelming (MacIntosh, 1988).

13. Has an Independent Component Completed in Advance

The ideal performance evaluation process allows for the two parties to come together and share their respective observations and conclusions. This meeting should occur at a time of mutual convenience and in a setting where neither evaluator nor evaluatee will be disturbed. Prior to this meeting, there should be a time when the employee and the supervisor have had an opportunity to score the performance evaluation instrument privately and independently. The parties can then come together, with responses initially determined, to share and discuss results.

This frequently does not occur in performance evaluation. In many instances, the evaluation is one-sided and the person being evaluated is simply provided the results. He/she may then be invited to respond but even this is not always the case.

Some performance evaluation procedures suggest joint assessment as a compromise to the sole assessment by superiors. Joint assessment can contain elements of duress and subtle pressures to compromise, and does not allow the more pensive self-reflection available through individual self-assessment. Furthermore, joint assessment at the time of review wastes time with scoring and marking evaluation forms that is better spent in dialogue about consensus or differences.

A fair and egalitarian approach to evaluation requires the opportunity for employees to evaluate themselves independently (Lombardi, 1988; MacIntosh, 1988; Rasmussen, 1988). Timmreck (1989) supports the position that any good evaluation system requires self-assessment as a fundamental component.

14. Is Non-Adversarial and Allows for Disagreement

A good performance evaluation instrument does not demand consensus. The parties need not come to agreement about raw scores on individual dimensions of the instrument. The individuals involved can, in fact, agree to disagree, and the subsequent dialogue about the disagreement can become the substance of the evaluation process. However, consensus and agreement needs to be reached in the areas of goal-setting and future planning.

The evaluation process should be non-competitive (Timmreck, 1989). By making the scoring the background for dialogue rather than the arena for argument, there is reduced pressure for concurrence, and a shift toward a more positive focus in the performance evaluation process. Reducing the discussion about scores and permitting individuals to disclose their own opinions allows attention to be focused on a more constructive task–a dialogue about what the instrument scores reflect in terms of their similarity or disparity, as well as goal setting for the future.

15. Is Responsive to Both Development and Diminution in Ability Over Time

An ideal performance evaluation instrument should be able to measure both growth and loss of function. It should also be able to demonstrate that an employee has hit a "plateau." Most instruments are designed to reflect continual upward movement over time. Employees expect that each evaluation will bring improved scores. This occurs in part because most appraisal instruments are constructed in such a way that the bottom step on a scale is the lowest level of organizational expectation and the top step is the highest. This "administratively driven" instrument then, through its construction, communicates at least implicitly that a person starts at the bottom and works his/her way up–somewhat like he/she does on the pay scale. To stop climbing the scale is akin to failure and falling on the scale runs the risk of experiencing administrative sanction and/or penalty. This is amplified, of course, if the performance evaluation is tied to raises or bonuses.

The assumption inherent in most performance evaluation instruments is that people always continue to improve. This, of course, is not the way things happen and is not an accurate reflection of reality. People do not always continue to improve. Some people "plateau" at a modest level of achievement. Others, during a particular review period and for reasons both personal and professional, do not perform at levels they had in the past.

An employee should not be expected to grow on every dimension every year. This is an unfortunate attitude communicated in most appraisal systems and we are vigorously opposed to it. Employees need to know that they can grow and develop but they can also "stay put." Our goals and aspirations, our commitment to our jobs, the priorities in our lives, all change throughout our work career. There are periods when we question what we are doing, when we feel "burned-out," when we need to pause for some "re-fueling." Perhaps we decide for a period of time to stop working through our lunch hour and train for a marathon instead. Perhaps we decide to pass up weekend workshops and other training activities to coach our daughter's soccer team. A performance evaluation system needs to have the flexibility to reflect these changes while at the same time setting a minimal expectation of performance.

The ideal instrument allows for a demonstration of growth, or stability, as well as loss of function. The use of the benchmark concept is critical here. By using the benchmark, the organization's expectation is made clear. Above the benchmark, the scale is concerned with professional growth and development and loss of function or "plateauing" in this area has little impact on organizational expectations.

In this sense, the ideal instrument is very robust. It allows people to move up and down the scale without impacting the organizational standards or expectations. If an individual's scores fall from the professional growth and development steps of the scale (for example, from step six back to step four), there is no reason for organizational concern. The expected organizational standard (the benchmark) is still being achieved. Furthermore, if the score remains at step four (the benchmark) for several review periods (across a three-year time period, for example), there is no organizational consequence because expected standards are being reached. In fact, the message that this approach communicates to employees is that it is perfectly acceptable to maintain a "steady state" once the benchmark has been achieved.

16. Is Available Immediately Upon Employment as Well as Throughout an Individual's Employment

When new employees are hired, they should immediately be made familiar with the evaluation instrument. The process of evaluation should be a standard part of the organization's orientation for new employees. The new employee's supervisor should spend time with him/her to review the instrument and outline its purpose and the various features and strengths–most especially, the aspects of positive, non-punitive style, professional growth features, and job-specific as well as generic aspects. Additionally, the individual should be oriented toward the first evaluation date and they should be encouraged to try out the instrument and bring any questions forward before that date. This early introduction to the review process increases employee comfort and reduces the chance for surprise on the evaluation date (Rasmussen, 1988; Spano, 1981; Timmreck, 1989).

17. Has High Content Validity

The performance evaluation instrument should "stay within its cover." In other words, everything that is relevant or expected through the evaluation is addressed by the instrument itself. The language should be the language of work and the dimensions involved should be self-explanatory (Dipboye and de Pontbriand, 1981). Much of this, as noted previously, is accomplished by utilizing employees in instrument construction (Schwab, Heneman, and DeCotiis, 1975).

18. Generates a Sense of Fairness

The ideal performance evaluation system should always appear fair and just to employees. The staff member's feedback should be that regardless of the results of the evaluation, the process was not suspect, and the instrument reflected both specific job duties and the generic aspects of human service work. Employee attitudes to the system of appraisal and its apparent "justice" can be as relevant as more traditional considerations of whether the instrument and process were valid or reliable (Bernardin and Beatty, 1984; Caroll and Schneier, 1982). Evans and McShane (1988) argue that "employee acceptance of appraisal decision outcomes depends at least partly upon their belief that observed characteristics of the performance appraisal system are consistent with fair process" (p. 178). Folger and Greenberg (1985) and Greenberg (1986) echo this sentiment. Such beliefs about the fairness and/or accuracy of the appraisal system are thought to influence employee motivation. Additionally, these attitudes toward the appraisal system might influence other more subtle outcomes such as organizational commitment and turnover (DeMarco and Nigro, 1983).

19. Is a Personalized Experience

Each employee should experience an individual flavor to the evaluation (Beer 1981; Spano, 1981). Such an experience requires that evaluations are not "group based" or made in comparison to fellow employees. It demands that the evaluatee has a chance to meet face to face to respond to his/her supervisor's ratings and that the individual has a chance for a self-appraisal. Failure to personalize the evaluation process in this fashion can lead to a loss of confidence and feelings of indifference, cynicism, and even hostility in the system (Wexley and Yukl, 1977).

20. Has a Goal Orientation Step as a Part of Closure

Toward the close of the evaluation process, discussion should focus on the future and, at the end of the instrument itself, there should be a section for a specification of goals and objectives for the future (Bechman, 1981). This is an open-ended section where both employee and supervisor respond. This component can begin with the independent appraisal of both employee and supervisor. Each party completes the goals and future planning section and returns for the joint interview where they share, try to reach a consensus on the key points, and sign off on the evaluation document. This is an important aspect of any ideal performance evaluation instrument (Burke, Wetzel, and Weir, 1978; Nemeroff and Wexley, 1979). There is a need for consensus at the closure of the evaluation process, and the goal orientation step is fundamental to this closure. This goal setting and the use of a standard criterion for measuring goal achievement, enhances the employee's belief in the objectivity of the appraisal results (Dipboye and de Pontbriand, 1981; Landy, Barnes, and Murphy, 1978).

21. One Instrument Fits All Staff

An ideal performance appraisal instrument should be usable by all staff, including management (Spano, 1981). The performance evaluation tool should have, as already mentioned, enough scope to include job-related and generic aspects. If this is the case, no one should be excluded by the instrument. This concept allows for unity around the instrument as well as a sense of loyalty. Staff know that the executive team is evaluated on the same core dimensions as they are. Each employee's job description is reflected in the total pool of dimensions, as are the generic human service expectations. Some dimensions become universal and are applied to everyone in the agency–no matter where he/she fits in the organizational hierarchy. These are the CORE dimensions. Other dimensions are applicable only to specific job groups. These are the À LA CARTE dimensions.

22. Can Grow and Change with the Agency

This "one size fits all staff" type of instrument can have the capacity to adapt to the growth or contraction of an organization. Because of this feature, the tool does not have to be rebuilt when new services are begun or discontinued. The ease and simplicity of this is extremely attractive. As an organization develops new services, all that is necessary is to meet with the job group to review existing dimensions of the instrument and select those appropriate to the new roles. Anything absent can be noted and subsequently built and added to the pool of dimensions available within the instrument. The generic dimensions are universal and will be part of the performance evaluation along with those selected from the existing pool. The newly constructed dimensions, built specifically for the employees delivering the new service, can be added to the existing pool.

A performance evaluation instrument that has such flexibility and an almost infinite range is invaluable. The instrument is designed around the position and not the particular staff member and can have extensive utility. It can grow with the agency and can be used with a broad range of roles and responsibilities.

23. Instrument is Comprised of Both Semantic and Numerical Components

An ideal performance evaluation tool requires descriptive features at each scale point. This means that each dimension is anchored with behavioral statements at each point on the scale. Each of these behavioral statements requires a numerical symbol that serves as a shorthand for an individual's location on a scale. This aids in discussion about ratings. These statements must be in clear and concise language that is descriptive of expected behavior. The supervisor or employee may be required during the evaluation to return to the exact statements on the dimension that led them to a particular score.

The numbers provide a way of quickly noticing and reviewing the dimensions. A system of numbers at each point on the scale allows the supervisor or employee to transfer the ratings onto a scoring grid for a view of the overall picture. Bechman (1981), as well as Landy and Farr (1983), advocate this combination of numerical ratings and substantiating comments as the most satisfactory performance evaluation design.

Chapter 4

Constructing the Ideal
Performance Evaluation Instrument
for a Human Service Agency

In this chapter the reader's attention is directed to the construction of the ideal performance evaluation instrument and implementation of the process. In building the instrument, the characteristics described in the previous chapter will be drawn upon and utilized. All of the characteristics described in Chapter 3 will be operationalized in a somewhat different order, reflecting the temporal sequence of instrument construction and system implementation.

INSTRUMENT CHARACTERISTICS

We advocate both semantic and numerical components to the evaluation instrument (Characteristic 23) and the most efficient method of meeting these expectations is through the use of behaviorally anchored rating scales (BARS).

The development of BARS was prompted largely by dissatisfaction with trait-based rating scales and by the realization that rating scales needed to be clarified for users by anchoring the various scale points with context-specific and job-related statements (Atkin and Conlon, 1978; Ferris, 1982; Schwab, Heneman, and DeCotiis, 1975). Such scales were first introduced by Smith and Kendall (1963) to evaluate the performance of nurses. The procedures used to develop the scale represented a variation and enhancement of the critical incident technique described by Flanagan (1954, p. 327):

> The critical incident technique consists of procedures . . . for collecting observed incidents having special significance and

meeting systematically defined criteria . . . . By an incident is meant any observable human activity that is sufficiently complete in itself to permit inferences and predictions to be made about the person performing the act. To be critical, an incident must occur in a situation where its consequences are sufficiently definite to leave little doubt concerning its effects.

Flanagan (1954, p. 327) emphasized that the technique was comprised of a flexible set of principles rather than a "single, rigid set of rules governing data collecting." Hence, the technique could be modified for a variety of practical applications.

Unlike the critical incident technique, Smith and Kendall (1963, p. 151) used "inferences or predictions (of behavior) from observations rather than actual observed behaviors." The format of the BARS developed by Smith and Kendall consisted of a set of continuous graphic rating scales arranged vertically on a page. Behavioral descriptions served as anchor points and were placed beside the numbers on the scale. Raters were instructed to check anywhere along the continuum. The rationale for the format was that it was perceived to be a "means of combining the relevance of direct observation of critical incidents and similar techniques with the acceptability to raters of graphic rating scales" (Smith and Kendall, 1963, p. 150).

Smith and Kendall (1963) noted that because such scales were referenced to behaviors, involved the actual raters or participants who were comparable to the actual raters, and included terminology germane to the raters, valid and conscientious ratings tended to result from their use.

An ideal instrument is one that can be utilized in the same way by everyone in the organization–from executive director to front-line worker (Characteristic 21). This implies that the instrument must, at some point, include dimensions which encompass and reflect every job description in the agency. Furthermore, both job specific and generic dimensions of human service work should be included (Characteristic 3). This means that the finished product should include dimensions specific to each job description (À LA CARTE) and generic (CORE) dimensions which are more agency, or human service based.

The reader will recall that a "benchmark" level of organizational expectation (Characteristic 4) is central to our performance evaluation system. It is this benchmark which provides the division between the administrative and professional development components of the dimensions. On the 7-point scale, there should be a step where the performance expectations, from the employer's perspective, reach a ceiling. Since the instrument is also concerned with professional growth and development (Characteristic 2), it should be apparent that the administrative ceiling of job expectations cannot go as far as point seven–otherwise, there would be no room to measure professional growth. The instrument must also be able to measure both development and loss of function (Characteristic 15). This means that the benchmark must be placed in such a way that it not only allows for professional growth components but also allows for some indication of a loss of ability when an evaluation warrants this consideration.

The choice of step four on the scale as the highest administrative expectation for performance on any dimension meets these various requirements. This allows three remaining steps to be directed solely towards professional growth and development. Additionally, if the semantic component of step four (its behavioral description, or expectation) is made a neutral statement that reflects the basic performance expectation, it allows three steps in the opposite direction for administrative concerns or a potential loss of function.

In review, we have a universally responsive instrument (Characteristic 21), consisting of job-specific and generic dimensions (Characteristic 3), using 7-step BARS-type scaling (Characteristic 23). It has a benchmark step for administrative expectations at step four (Characteristic 4) which allows for three upper steps of self-development and professional growth (Characteristic 2) and three lower steps of administrative demand, and which allows for a consideration of the loss of ability over time (Characteristic 15).

INSTRUMENT CONSTRUCTION
WITH STAFF PARTICIPATION

Employee commitment and participation in the construction of the performance evaluation instrument is fundamental to its success. Without it, there is little merit in pursuing the process. This should begin with a general staff meeting, where the project is communicated to all involved parties. Questions can be fielded about the few decisions that have been made to this point (choice of type of instrument scaling, benchmark separation of administrative and professional growth elements, for example). Above all else, what needs to be communicated is that the intent of management is sincere and the purposes of the performance evaluation are both organizational *and* individual growth and the promotion of a professional attitude toward evaluation and work. It needs to be emphasized at this meeting that the process is not to be associated with pay, or other financial rewards (Characteristic 5).

This is a controversial issue in performance evaluation and employees may need to have clarification and reassurance on this point. Time should be set aside to reassure skeptical employees that management is serious about disconnecting evaluation from monetary issues. The aim of the general staff meeting, then, is to gain support for the project and to seek employee participation.

Subsequent meetings can then take place in job groups and should begin with a review of the information from the earlier general staff meeting. The effort at this point is to proceed with a commitment to begin the process of identifying job dimensions. These dimensions are those which are considered to discretely concern a specific job group and their particular role and service in the agency. At this stage, it is only a general description of the job dimensions that is required.

After specific job groups have met and identified job dimensions, these dimensions are pooled across all job groups. Invariably, there will be dimensions in common. These dimensions may have different titles, but upon review, it is clear that they are describing the same expectations across different jobs, roles, and service responsibilities. In other words, they are generic to work in any capacity within that particular organization. On the other hand, the job groups will also identify dimensions of work which pertain only to them.

The outcome of this exercise, in addition to fostering a commitment to building their own performance evaluation instrument, is the identification of both job specific (À LA CARTE) and generic (CORE) expectations required of employees in the organization.

The next task for the job groups is to construct the performance evaluation scale for each À LA CARTE dimension. The reader will recall that each of these scales will consist of seven steps with a behavioral description for each step. The first four steps can be derived from the job description with the fourth step a neutral statement reflecting achievement of the expectation. The next three steps beyond step four are behavioral statements which reflect aspects of professional growth and development related to this dimension. These steps are considered as beyond the basic job description, or above any minimal administrative expectation.

It is not easy to build such a performance evaluation scale. For example, it must be non-punitive and positive (Characteristic 1), and use commonly understood, simple language (Characteristic 6). The non-punitive, positive aspect is addressed to some extent by the fact that only four steps of the 7-step scale are administratively-driven. This allows for three steps dedicated to professional growth issues. Our experience is that it is exceedingly difficult to avoid the "jargon" and buzzwords of the professions involved in human service work (social work, psychology, etc.). Nevertheless, a "screening" is absolutely necessary if one wishes to build an instrument that is clearly understood and free of the potential for different interpretations or distortion.

The "ideal" performance evaluation instrument also requires expectations to be anchored in real situations and be readily understood by anyone evaluated on the dimension (Characteristic 8). This may not be difficult for the first four steps because each job group can return for guidance to the actual job description. The last three steps, however, require more thought and effort and will rely heavily upon the experience and leadership of key people in the job group who can describe the principal aspects of professional growth and development with respect to a particular job dimension.

The second set of dimensions are the CORE dimensions–those that are considered universal and generic to all employees in the organization. We recommend that these scales be constructed by a small cross-section of job group representatives who will define the dimensions and identify the seven behavioral anchors. As with the

À LA CARTE dimensions each has seven steps, with the first four steps grounded in the job description and administrative expectations. The fourth step is a neutral statement of the basic expectation and the last three steps are concerned with professional growth and development.

The orientation of all dimensions, whether CORE or À LA CARTE, should be toward the future and toward tomorrow's employee (Characteristic 11). As noted already, the dimensions are positive in intention and tone (Characteristic 1), and are written in simple, clearly understood language (Characteristic 6). They are constructed through staff participation (Characteristic 7), and they are not tied to pay, or merit increases (Characteristic 5).

The resulting instrument consists of a set of CORE dimensions and another of À LA CARTE dimensions. The number of À LA CARTE scales is virtually unlimited and depends on the number and diversity of programs within a particular organization. A final task for each job group is to reach agreement with management on which À LA CARTE dimensions will be used with their particular group.

The process can be tiring and time consuming. Indeed, a recurring criticism of BARS-type evaluation instruments is the time and expense involved in instrument construction (Cronbach, 1970; Thorndike and Hagen, 1977). However, we argue that the outcome is well worth the effort. Most of us have learned that it is wise to practice preventive maintenance on the vehicles we drive ("Pay me a little now, or pay me much more later!"). In similar fashion, the future costs of not having a well-developed performance evaluation system–through employee turnover, lowered productivity, poor morale, possible litigation–more than justifies the "front-end" expense.

THE PERFORMANCE EVALUATION PROCESS

Returning to our list of characteristics of the "ideal" performance evaluation instrument and process, the reader is reminded that the process should be fast and efficient (Characteristic 12) and have an independent component (Characteristic 13). Additionally, there must be opportunity for dialogue and disagreement (Characteristic 14), and the process must be time-framed and repetitive (Characteristic 9).

To illustrate the performance evaluation process in action, let us assume that an organization has completed the tasks of dimension identification and scale construction. The resulting instrument consists of ten CORE dimensions and another 22 À LA CARTE dimensions. Through negotiation and agreement with management, a particular job group (e.g., residential staff) has ten of these À LA CARTE dimensions designated as part of its evaluation. This group, then, will be evaluated by using 20 scales, the ten CORE dimensions and the ten agreed upon À LA CARTE dimensions.

The evaluation of a particular residential staff member would begin with two independent processes. The worker would score himself/herself on each 7-point scale (20 scales in all) and the worker's supervisor would do likewise. Our experience is that this is not an onerous or time-consuming task and should not take more than one hour for either person to complete.

Once this independent component is completed, the next step is a face-to-face meeting between supervisor and staff member. We can not stress enough the importance of dedicating this time exclusively to the performance evaluation. We speak here, particularly, to the supervisor. Nothing is more frustrating or vexing for an employee than to have his or her evaluation interrupted by telephone calls or other diversions. Not only does it detract from the event, it communicates a clear message that the employee and his/her evaluation are not important to the supervisor.

The purpose of this meeting is to share scores and to engage in dialogue about them. The need for clear and open communication at this meeting is critical. It should be made clear that disagreement is perfectly acceptable. While either party can feel free to change scores because of discussion, new information, clarification, and so forth, there should be no requirement that people arrive at a consensus. Employee and supervisor can agree to disagree and each are "allowed" to retain their own set of scores. This understanding reduces animosity and pressure toward consensus. It promotes a sense of justice and fairness in the employee about the process (Characteristic 18).

The only criterion which must be respected is that people defend their scoring on the basis of the actual behavioral description contained within the performance evaluation scale (Characteristic 17). The scores must be based upon that data and not on subjective impressions, personalities, or on the basis of one or two critical incidents.

A second face-to-face meeting is recommended two weeks after the above meeting. At this meeting, the focus should be on goals and objectives for the coming year. This requires a summary sheet be included as part of the performance evaluation instrument. It allows for comments about the process, a delineation of goals and objectives, and a place for employee and supervisor to sign off (Characteristic 20).

This step provides closure to the evaluation process. At this point, both parties should feel that there are no "loose strings" or unfinished business. Both employee and supervisor have said all that needed to be said and the final consideration is about tomorrow, and about potential growth and career development. While the individuals are not required to agree on scores, there should be some consensus about goals and objectives. While time lengths may vary, our experience is that the entire process–independent scoring, face-to-face meeting about scores, and face-to-face meeting about goals, objectives, and sign-off–should not exceed three hours.

The independent component, the face-to-face meeting, and the willingness to "live with disagreement" all serve to personalize and individualize the performance evaluation process (Characteristic 19). The utilization of the À LA CARTE feature is also critical to this process in that each employee has had input into the decision of which factors will be included in his/her evaluation.

Once the instrument has been implemented and found successful, it should become a part of the orientation package for new employees (Characteristic 16) and become an integral part of organizational policy and procedure. Employees should be encouraged to read it and bring forward their concerns. New employees are informed of the process, their evaluation dates are agreed upon, and agreement is reached on the À LA CARTE dimensions which will be included in their review. If the position is a new one or is part of a new program, the new employee will need to be engaged in scale construction with the supervisor to develop a dimension (or dimensions) to be included in the À LA CARTE group of scales. This early introduction of new employees to their responsibility in helping to build the performance evaluation system fosters loyalty and commitment to it.

The CORE and À LA CARTE features of this system allow it to change with the organization and provide it with tremendous flexibility (Characteristic 22). As new programs are developed or introduced, the À LA CARTE dimensions are expanded. As programs are abandoned, the À LA CARTE dimensions used to evaluate performance in them can be discarded.

An added strength of the performance evaluation system described here is the User's Guide (Characteristic 10) which becomes a part of the instrument. The User's Guide reviews the purposes of the performance evaluation system, the BARS-type scaling that is used, and provides a definition of each dimension. The User's Guide is of great assistance to employees–particularly new ones– and it can reduce the potential for disagreement between supervisor and employee.

The construction of the performance evaluation instrument and the implementation of the process is now complete. We have a universal instrument which has both job-specific and generic dimensions and is built with semantic and numerical aspects. Furthermore, it has a benchmark, it emphasizes professional growth and development, is not tied to pay, or incentives, and it allows for growth in, or loss of, ability over time. The instrument and procedures were built with employee participation, and the system is positive and non-punitive in intent.

The instrument uses clear and simple language that is devoid of jargon and "buzzwords" and describes expectations that are grounded in the real experience of employees who do the work. It is directed at the future and not the past, and has high content validity. It is fast and efficient and while requiring the interactive participation of all parties at some points, also allows for an independent component as well. Participants are allowed to disagree, experience a sense of fairness and openness, and an appreciation that the process was personalized. It is time-framed and repetitive and is introduced immediately upon employment as part of new employee orientation.

If the process which has been described in this chapter is followed, a performance evaluation system which embodies all 23 characteristics will result. To repeat what was said earlier, this process takes time and effort and is labor-intensive. However, a failure to work through this process is to invite the common problems and failings of the majority of performance evaluation models.

Chapter 5

The Performance Evaluation Instrument

Now that the reader has an understanding of the characteristics of the "ideal" performance evaluation instrument and the method of construction, a complete instrument is presented in this chapter. It was developed by the authors for a child and adolescent service agency in northeastern Ontario, Canada. Each of the 23 characteristics is either present in the instrument itself, or is employed in the process.

To fully illustrate the advocated model the instrument is presented in its entirety as it would be provided to an employee. It contains the complete set of CORE and À LA CARTE scales, the User's Guide, and the Sign-Off form. This instrument was developed by a particular agency for application with a particular set of job functions; hence it would not be advisable to attempt to lift this instrument directly for use in another setting. A valid, reliable, and employee-responsive performance evaluation system can only be developed by adhering to the process described in the previous chapter and tailoring the result to the specific agency.

CONTENTS

1. Introduction
2. The Scale
3. The Dimensions
4. Time Boundaries
5. The Wording of the Dimensions
6. The Evaluation Process
7. Goal Setting Component of the Process
8. Performance Evaluation Instrument:

CORE DIMENSION A:
Establishment and Maintenance of Cooperative Relationships
with Colleagues

CORE DIMENSION B:
Understanding and Maintaining of Relationships with Other
Relevant Organizations

CORE DIMENSION C:
Knowledge of the Characteristics of the Target Population

CORE DIMENSION D:
Awareness and Relevance of the Organization's Policies
and Services to the Problems of the Target Population

CORE DIMENSION E:
Interpretation of the Organization to the Public

CORE DIMENSION F:
Knowledge and Use of Community Resources

CORE DIMENSION G:
Awareness and Commitment to Professional Values and Ethics

CORE DIMENSION H:
Responsibility for Individual Professional Development

CORE DIMENSION I:
Organization of Work and Time Management

CORE DIMENSION J:
Appropriate Use of Consultation and Supervision

CORE DIMENSION K:
Utilization and Provision of Organizationally Based
Opportunities for Staff Development

À LA CARTE DIMENSION L:
Establishment and Maintenance of a Professional Relationship
with Clients

À LA CARTE DIMENSION M:
Problem Identification and Assessment

À LA CARTE DIMENSION N:
Identification of Alternative Courses of Clinical Disposition
and Selection of an Intervention Plan

À LA CARTE DIMENSION O:
Implementation and Evaluation of an Intervention Plan

À LA CARTE DIMENSION P:
Provision of an External Consultative Service

À LA CARTE DIMENSION Q:
Ability to Demonstrate Oral and Written Communication Skills

À LA CARTE DIMENSION R:
Applied Knowledge of Child/Adolescent Care

À LA CARTE DIMENSION S:
Ability to Work as Part of a Team

À LA CARTE DIMENSION T:
Management of Human Resources

À LA CARTE DIMENSION U:
Program Planning, Development, and Evaluation

À LA CARTE DIMENSION V:
Fiscal/Budget Planning and Management

À LA CARTE DIMENSION W:
Agency Advocacy and Service Integration

À LA CARTE DIMENSION X:
Coordination of Client Services

À LA CARTE DIMENSION Y:
Ability to Demonstrate Office Practice Skills

9. Performance Evaluation Instrument Score Sheet
10. Comments

INTRODUCTION

This performance evaluation instrument was developed in response to the need to evaluate staff on an annual basis. Staff evaluation is as essential for professional development, and for personal growth and individual goal setting, as it is valuable in establishing the criteria for effective performance. This instrument is designed to reflect both aspects of service: personal growth and effective performance.

Added to the focus of this instrument is the consideration of two other important areas. These are: (a) the general professional expectations of any human service role, and (b) the specific areas defined by individual job descriptions.

To address these specific elements of work, the instrument is divided into two sections. One is considered the generic aspect and the dimensions are termed "CORE DIMENSIONS." The second is more specific to a particular job description and the dimensions are considered "À LA CARTE."

To respond effectively each and every person would reply to the CORE DIMENSIONS and also respond to those À LA CARTE dimensions which had been pre–selected and accepted by his/her job group.

The intention of the tool is to promote professional growth, and to provide a benchmark for evaluation against an established criterion. The procedure is to respond to all the CORE DIMENSIONS, and the pre-selected À LA CARTE dimensions which are specific to your job description.

THE SCALE

The dimensions are given titles which delineate the essence of the particular job expectation. Each dimension is broken down into seven steps of performance. Each step on the seven-point scale contains a descriptive statement of the performance at that step.

Each seven-point scale has a criterion, or benchmark, of performance. The benchmark is always considered as the fourth (four) step of the scale. This step four is a neutral statement which reflects the expected level of performance for any employee on that dimension. Any level of response below four is considered less than expected performance, while any score above four reflects more than expected performance.

When responding to the scale it is suggested that you initially read step four. If you can respond favorably to step four then read step five. If you respond favorably to step five then move to step six. The same process applies if you respond unfavorably to step four. The attempt is to be honest and reach a step on the scale which accurately corresponds to your current level of performance.

The employee responds to the instrument independently and the designated supervisor, clinical director, or administrator, also completes the process independently. It should be kept in mind that although every dimension has a seven-point scale, and step four is always the benchmark, the flow of the scales is not always a progression from one through seven. Sometimes it will appear that there is a shift from step four to step five, or from step five to step six. This should not be a matter for concern or anxiety. Any step beyond four reflects professional growth, or a display of clinical acumen, and this demands that the scale show an expansion of expectation. You will find then, that the steps from one to four are linear and progress comfortably, while steps four through seven will usually do this, but not on every dimension.

THE DIMENSIONS

The dimensions are more than titles, and the key to a successful reply to the instrument is to objectively consider the statement at each step of the scale. Each dimension, however, has been selected because it is unique and is not replicated anywhere else in the instrument. Each dimension stands alone and should not be blended or confused with any other dimension. Dimensions that deal with clinical issues should not be confused with procedure dimensions. Dimensions that deal with colleagues should not be confused with those that deal with clients. Consider each dimension singularly and try to confine your thinking to the content of the statements. Do not read things into the content. Do not try to imagine what is really meant! Do not go beyond the evident focus of the dimension.

TIME BOUNDARIES

When you respond to the instrument keep in mind that it is concerned with a period of time. If you use the instrument every six months then it should reflect the past six months and not the lifetime of your work with the agency or institution. If it is done yearly it should consider the whole year, and not just last week, or last month. This means that one error or one success is not the key to your response to step four, or step five, and so on.

The key to your response should be the overall ability, or pattern of behavior you have displayed in the past six months, or one year, depending on your particular organization's time frame for evaluation.

THE WORDING OF THE DIMENSIONS

Effort has been made to eliminate categorical words like always, every, often, never. All the words cannot be eliminated, however, so there will be occasions when you will become "reactive" to a word. Try to stay within the intent of the instrument and seek patterns and styles across time. Try not to seize upon single incidents, or a particular critical event. Occasionally these events are relevant to make a point about style or pattern, but for the most part these "reactive" words should be treated with less power than they could generate.

THE EVALUATION PROCESS

Usually each person does the scoring independently and the designated individuals come together to share their evaluations. It is hoped that there would be reasonable consensus on most of the scores for each dimension. It is common to differ by one score in either direction and this is not an issue. If differences exist that are greater than one step on any dimension it should serve as an opportunity to dialogue about the dimension. Sometimes the differences are a result of misunderstanding the intent of the dimension, or the wording of the step. More often the disagreement is genuine resulting in professional dialogue and the opportunity for goal setting.

The purpose of the process is not to reach consensus. It is not expected that individuals reach agreement on the "right" score. It is expected that there is honest effort to communicate about the scores and the reasons behind them.

People are allowed to agree and to disagree. If individuals wish to move scores as a result of the dialogue and the evaluation process it is perfectly appropriate to do so. If they do not wish to move their score this is also appropriate. The tool is designed for feedback, education, supervision, goal setting, and professional development. It is not an instrument that has any punitive intent and should not be used in association with any pay, promotion, or increment salary. Response should be positive and open-minded.

GOAL SETTING COMPONENT OF THE PROCESS

After completing the independent scoring, and the face-to-face meetings, there should be an opportunity to return to the process for the last component–goal setting and sign-off. This element of the protocol is suggested to occur approximately two weeks after the evaluation process. Each participant provides comments and attempts to find agreed-upon goals and objectives that will serve as guidelines for the coming year and which will be reconsidered at the next scheduled evaluation meeting. A summary sheet is provided to assist the participants in this component of the process. The staff member provides comments about the previous step of the process, independent evaluation, and face-to-face meeting, as does the designated supervisor(s).

It should be understood that the involved players do not complete the comment and goal-setting sheets until after the two earlier steps are accomplished. The comments should reflect the appreciations or concerns of the process; and the goals should consider the content of the face-to-face meeting. For these reasons it is important to complete this final step when all the information about the process is available and particularly relevant. Once again, it must be remembered that the process is intended to be positive, objective, and constructive. The comments section should be honest and frank, and the goals should be mutually acceptable.

PERFORMANCE EVALUATION INSTRUMENT

CORE DIMENSION A:

Establishment and Maintenance of Cooperative Relationships with Colleagues

This dimension has to do with work-related activity and not with outside social behaviour. It is concerned with how you deal with your colleagues within the employment setting. It is also confined to your behavior, and is not an attempt to evaluate the way others behave toward you. Try to respond to this dimension in terms of how you relate, at work, with your professional colleagues.

7. This person cooperates with colleagues in a way that continually demonstrates helpful, supportive, and respectful collegial relationships.
6. This person cooperates with colleagues, provides support, and demonstrates respectful relationships.
5. This person cooperates with colleagues and assumes responsibility for providing professional support to these colleagues.

4. THIS PERSON COOPERATES WITH COLLEAGUES WITH RESPECT TO THEIR MUTUAL ROLES AND RESPONSIBILITIES.

3. This person can cooperate with colleagues but his/her behavior may fail to respect their mutual roles and responsibilities.
2. This person has difficulty cooperating with colleagues and fails to respect their mutual roles and responsibilities.
1. This person is unable to cooperate with colleagues and is disrespectful within their mutual roles and responsibilities.

CORE DIMENSION B:

Understanding and Maintaining Relationships with Other Relevant Organizations

This dimension addresses organizations outside your agency. The dimension is asking whether you feel your work appropriately reflects an understanding of your agency's administrative protocols and mandate. This concerns only those agencies which have ongoing relationships with yours, and with whom you should be familiar and actively engaged.

7. This person comprehensively understands the mandate and administrative protocols of the agency, knows and appreciates how these agency operations relate to other relevant organizations, and can assist in the development and maintenance of these operations.

6. This person completely understands the mandate and administrative protocols of the agency, knows and appreciates how these agency operations relate to other relevant organizations, and can assist in the maintenance of these operations.

5. This person clearly understands the mandate and administrative protocols of the agency, and knows and appreciates how these agency operations relate to other relevant organizations.

4. THIS PERSON UNDERSTANDS THE MANDATE AND ADMINISTRATIVE PROTOCOLS OF THE AGENCY, AND KNOWS HOW THESE AGENCY OPERATIONS RELATE TO OTHER RELEVANT ORGANIZATIONS.

3. This person has some understanding of the mandate and administrative protocols of the agency, and knows to some extent how these agency operations relate to other relevant organizations.

2. This person is limited in his/her understanding of the mandate and administrative protocols of the agency, and has restricted knowledge of how these agency operations relate to other relevant organizations.

1. This person is ignorant of the mandate and administrative protocols of the agency, and does not know how these agency operations relate to other relevant organizations.

CORE DIMENSION C:

Knowledge of the Characteristics of the Target Population

This dimension addresses your knowledge and understanding of the target population being addressed, or served by your agency. Do you adequately demonstrate an awareness and appreciation of the type of difficulties or problems the target group experiences?

7. This person demonstrates a detailed and comprehensive appreciation of the characteristics of the target population. He/she can specify and appreciate the major problems the target group is experiencing, is sensitive to shifts and changes in this service population, and can utilize this sensitivity in anticipating service needs.

6. This person demonstrates a detailed and comprehensive knowledge of the characteristics of the target population. He/she can specify and appreciate the major problems the target group is experiencing, and is sensitive to shifts and changes in this service population.

5. This person demonstrates a detailed knowledge of the characteristics of the target population. He/she can specify and appreciate the major problems the target group is experiencing.

4. THIS PERSON HAS KNOWLEDGE OF THE CHARACTERISTICS OF THE TARGET POPULATION. HE/SHE CAN SPECIFY THE MAJOR PROBLEMS THE TARGET GROUP IS EXPERIENCING.

3. This person can identify some characteristics of the target population and can specify some of the major problems the target group is experiencing, but he/she lacks a clear appreciation of the range of characteristics and problems.

2. This person has difficulty identifying the characteristics of the target population. He/She cannot readily specify the major problems the target group is experiencing.

1. This person is ignorant of the characteristics of the target population. He/she is unable to specify any of the problems the target group is experiencing.

CORE DIMENSION D:

Awareness and Relevance of the Organization's Policies and Services to the Problems of the Target Population

This dimension is concerned with your ability to understand and appreciate the policies, and/or services of your agency and, in doing so, to see how these "fit" the target population. The dimension asks if your understanding reflects an awareness of how policies and services address the target population.

7. This worker has a comprehensive awareness of organizational policies and services. He/she has a thorough appreciation of the purpose and relevance of these policies and services to the target population, and both initiates and participates in discussion which can lead to new policies and services.

6. This person has a comprehensive awareness of organizational policies and services. He/she can fully appreciate the purpose and relevance of these policies and services to the target population, and participates in discussion which can lead to new policies and/or services.

5. This person has a complete awareness of organization policies and/or services. He/she can fully appreciate the purpose and relevance of these policies and service to the target population.

4. THIS PERSON HAS AN AWARENESS OF ORGANIZATION POLICIES AND SERVICES. HE/SHE CAN APPRECIATE THE PURPOSE AND RELEVANCE OF THESE POLICIES AND SERVICES TO THE TARGET POPULATION.

3. This person has a limited awareness of organizational policies and services. He/she has a restricted appreciation of the purpose and relevance of these policies and services to the target population.

2. This person has little awareness of organizational policies and services. He/she appreciates only incidentally the purpose and relevance of these policies and services to the target population.

1. This person demonstrates an ignorance of organizational policies and services and a contempt for the purpose and relevance of these policies and services to the target population.

CORE DIMENSION E:

Interpretation of the Organization to the Public

This dimension considers your ability to interpret the organization to the general public. Do your actions respect the public's requests about your organization and its services? Are you able to respond reasonably to inquiries from interested persons and to do so appropriately?

7. This person can comfortably and accurately interpret the organization to the public. He/she can respond thoroughly to public requests in a supportive, non-defensive way, and respects the public's right to know about the organization and its services. He/she refers inquiries to the appropriate resource, uses consultation when necessary, and could represent the agency in any public presentation.

6. This person can comfortably interpret the organization to the public. He/she can respond thoroughly to public requests in a supportive, non-defensive way, and respects the public's right to know about the organization and its services. He/she refers inquiries to the appropriate resource and uses consultation when necessary.

5. This person can comfortably interpret the organization to the public. He/she can fully respond to public requests in a supportive, non-defensive way, and respects the public's right to know about the organization and its services.

4. | THIS PERSON CAN INTERPRET THE ORGANIZATION TO THE PUBLIC. HE/SHE RESPONDS TO PUBLIC REQUESTS IN A SUPPORTIVE WAY AND RESPECTS THE PUBLIC'S RIGHT TO KNOW ABOUT THE ORGANIZATION AND ITS SERVICES.

3. This person has difficulty interpreting the organization to the public. He/she responds to public requests with reservation and can fail to respect the public's right to know about the organization and its services.

2. This person is ineffective at interpreting the organization to the public. He/she responds to public requests with avoidance and

fails to respect the public's right to know about the organization and its services.

1. This person is unable to interpret the organization to the public. He/she responds to public requests with disdain, and is indifferent to the public's right to know about the organization and its services.

CORE DIMENSION F:

Knowledge and Use of Community Resources

This dimension is concerned with those community resources which impact on the target population. Do you have a knowledge of these resources and their specific expectations? Could you assist your client from an information base about these other resources?

7. This person has broad and extensive knowledge of community resources. He/she makes informed and responsive decisions about service based upon this knowledge. He/she is aware that individuals may have difficulty accessing these services and is willing to assist, and is conscious of the need to follow-up on this community initiative.

6. This person has broad knowledge of community resources. He/she makes informed and responsive decisions about service based upon this knowledge. He/she is aware that individuals may have difficulty accessing these services and is willing to assist.

5. This person has broad knowledge of community resources. He/she makes informed and responsive decisions about service based upon this knowledge.

4. THIS PERSON HAS KNOWLEDGE OF COMMUNITY RESOURCES. HE/SHE MAKES INFORMED DECISIONS ABOUT SERVICE BASED UPON THIS KNOWLEDGE.

3. This person has moderate knowledge of community resources. He/she makes reasonably informed decisions about service based on this knowledge.

2. This person has insufficient knowledge of community resources. He/she is unable to make decisions about service without assistance.

1. This person has a poverty of knowledge about community resources. He/she makes inappropriate decisions about service because of the absence of this knowledge.

CORE DIMENSION G:

Awareness and Commitment to Professional Values and Ethics

This dimension addresses both private and public behavior that is role related. It is not addressing behavior that is not role related. Do you act in an ethical manner? Do you know what the major ethical issues are? Are you committed to the practice of professional values and ethics?

7. This person is aware and mindful of the major values and ethical principles which apply to his/her role, and has a genuine commitment to the upholding of these principles. He/she has no difficulty implementing these principles and can demonstrate how these principles are applied in his/her practice.*

6. This person is aware and mindful of the major values and ethical principles which apply to his/her role, and has a genuine commitment to the upholding of these values. He/she has no difficulty implementing these principles in their professional role.

5. This person is aware and mindful of the major values and ethical principles which apply to his/her role, and has a genuine commitment to the upholding of these principles.

4. | THIS PERSON IS AWARE OF THE MAJOR VALUES AND ETHICAL PRINCIPLES WHICH APPLY TO HIS/HER ROLE (SUCH AS, CONFIDENTIALITY, INDIVIDUAL WORTH AND DIGNITY, INTEGRITY IN RELATIONSHIPS, RESPONSIBILITY TO SOCIETY . . .), AND HAS A COMMITMENT TO THE UPHOLDING OF THESE PRINCIPLES.

3. This person has moderate awareness of the major values and

---

* The major principles above have been drawn from the guidelines on professional standards and ethics of the American Psychological Association, Canadian Psychological Association, National Association of Social Workers, and Canadian Association of Social Workers.

ethical principles which apply to his/her role, and has an interest in the upholding of these principles.

2. This person has limited awareness of the major values and ethical principles which apply to his/her role, and has little interest in the upholding of these principles.

1. This person is contemptuous of the major values and ethical principles which apply to his/her role, and is disinterested in the upholding of these principles.

CORE DIMENSION H:

Responsibility for Individual Professional Development

This dimension is concerned with efforts to support your own professional development, and your commitment to this self-development. The dimension considers agency-supported activities, and should not be scored in consideration of private initiatives which are enhancing and show motivation, but do not directly reflect role-specific development.

7. This person accepts and welcomes responsibility for professional development. He/she demonstrates an enthusiastic commitment to such professional development, and regularly seeks and promotes opportunities for such development.
6. This person accepts and welcomes responsibility for professional development. He/she demonstrates an enthusiastic commitment to such development, and regularly seeks opportunities for such development.
5. This person accepts responsibility for professional development. He/she demonstrates an enthusiastic commitment to such development.

4. THIS PERSON ACCEPTS RESPONSIBILITY FOR PROFESSIONAL DEVELOPMENT. HE/SHE DEMONSTRATES A COMMITMENT TO SUCH DEVELOPMENT.

3. This person accepts some responsibility for professional development. He/she shows conditional commitment to such development and may find reason to excuse himself/herself when it is inconvenient or in competition with other activities.
2. This person takes minimal responsibility for professional development. He/she shows sporadic commitment to such development and commonly avoids such activity.
1. This person accepts no responsibility for professional development. He/she shows no commitment to such development.

CORE DIMENSION I:

Organization of Work and Time Management

This dimension examines the ability to organize your time and work. It does not talk about the quality of that work but of the organization and time management of the work itself. The quality of work is examined on other dimensions.

7. This person demonstrates superior organizational and time management skills, willingly offers support and assistance around these matters, and serves as a role model for others.
6. This person demonstrates excellent organizational and time management skills and willingly offers support and assistance around these matters.
5. This person is well organized in the work situation and is adept at managing his/her time.
4. THIS PERSON IS ABLE TO ORGANIZE HIS/HER WORK AND MANAGE HIS/HER TIME.
3. This person requires occasional supervision to organize his/her work and manage his/her time.
2. This person requires regular supervision to ensure that work is organized. Frequent reminders are required to ensure that tasks are completed on time.
1. This person requires constant supervision to ensure that work is organized and time frames are met.

CORE DIMENSION J:

Appropriate Use of Consultation and Supervision

This dimension considers your attitude and approach to consultation and supervision. Do you value consultation and supervision and utilize them in a professional manner? Do you make an effort to incorporate information received from consultation or supervision when it would be appropriate to do so? This dimension asks about your approach to supervision. It does not consider whether others provide good supervision or not, or whether they provide consultation or supervision in a helpful manner.

7. This person values and appropriately utilizes consultation and/or supervision. He/she astutely incorporates information that was reviewed and discussed, seeks clarification when additional information is required, and can integrate the associated themes and issues.

6. This person values and appropriately utilizes consultation and/or supervision. He/she astutely incorporates information that was reviewed and discussed, and seeks clarification when additional information is required.

5. This person appropriately utilizes consultation and/or supervision. He/she incorporates information that was reviewed and discussed, and seeks clarification when additional information is required.

4. THIS PERSON UTILIZES CONSULTATION AND/OR SUPERVISION. HE/SHE INCORPORATES INFORMATION THAT WAS REVIEWED AND DISCUSSED.

3. This person makes occasional use of consultation and/or supervision. He/she may incorporate information that was reviewed and discussed.

2. This person makes little use of consultation and/or supervision. He/she is indifferent about incorporating information that was reviewed or discussed.

1. This person does not utilize consultation and/or supervision. He/she is disinterested in incorporating anything that might be reviewed or discussed.

CORE DIMENSION K:

Utilization and Provision of Organizationally Based Opportunities for Staff Development

This dimension asks whether you make efforts to provide learning opportunities for your colleagues through available organization channels, such as inservice, or professional workshop days. If you do not provide such opportunities, do you attend, support and encourage these events or opportunities?

7. This person regularly provides organizationally based opportunities for staff development, actively encourages and supports for such opportunities for others, diligently attends and contributes, and serves as a role model for others in the promotion of this aspect of organizational development.
6. This person frequently provides organizationally based opportunities for staff development, actively encourages and supports such opportunities for others, and diligently attends and contributes.
5. This person is willing, and with encouragement will provide organizationally based opportunities for staff development, supports and fosters such opportunities for others, and regularly attends and contributes.

4. THIS PERSON PROVIDES ORGANIZATIONALLY BASED OPPORTUNITIES FOR STAFF DEVELOPMENT, SUPPORTS AND FOSTERS SUCH ACTIVITY IN OTHERS, AND REGULARLY ATTENDS AND CONTRIBUTES.

3. This person appreciates the need for the provision of organizationally based opportunities for staff development, supports or fosters such activity in others, but does not regularly attend or contribute.
2. This person has little appreciation for organizationally based opportunities for staff development, may support or foster this activity in others, but does not attend, or finds reasons to avoid attending.

1. This person has no interest in organizationally based opportunities for staff development, may even discourage others or hinder such activity, and will not attend unless required.

À LA CARTE DIMENSION L:

Establishment and Maintenance of a Professional Relationship with Clients

This dimension examines your appreciation of your role with clients. Can you separate your work role from your personal involvement? Can you establish boundaries and set schedules and goals? Are you able to create a professional distance between yourself and your clients?

7. This person is continually able to establish and maintain a professional relationship with clients. He/she completely understands and preserves the distinction between his/her professional role and that of personal conduct, and keeps and sustains relationships at a level of propriety.

6. This person is clearly able to establish and maintain a professional relationship with clients. He/she completely understands and appreciates the distinction between his/her professional role and that of personal conduct, and keeps and sustains relationships at a level of propriety.

5. This person is able to establish and maintain a professional relationship with clients. He/she completely understands the distinction between his/her professional role and that of personal conduct, and keeps relationships with clients at a level of propriety.

4. THIS PERSON IS ABLE TO ESTABLISH AND MAINTAIN A PROFESSIONAL RELATIONSHIP WITH CLIENTS. HE/SHE KNOWS THE DISTINCTION BETWEEN HIS/HER PROFESSIONAL ROLE AND THAT OF PERSONAL CONDUCT, AND KEEPS RELATIONSHIPS WITH CLIENTS AT A LEVEL OF PROPRIETY.

3. This person makes an effort to establish and maintain a professional relationship with clients. He/she is aware of the distinction between his/her professional role and that of personal conduct, and attempts to keep relationships with clients at a level of propriety.

2. This person has difficulty establishing and maintaining a professional relationship with clients. He/she loses sight of the distinction between his/her professional role and that of personal conduct, and can fail to keep relationships with clients at a level of propriety.

1. This person does not establish and maintain a professional relationship with clients. He/she neglects the distinction between his/her professional role and that of personal conduct, and fails to keep relationships with clients at a level of propriety.

À LA CARTE DIMENSION M:

Problem Identification and Assessment

This dimension considers your ability to identify and assess problems. Are you able to collect information and to prioritize the presenting problems? Can you see how these problems interfere with client functioning?

7. This person has a superior ability to collect data and identify significant client problems. He/she can expertly see how the problems interfere with client functioning.
6. This person has an excellent ability to collect data and identify significant client problems. He/she can skillfully see how the problems interfere with client functioning.
5. This person has advanced ability to collect data and identify significant client problems. He/she can readily see how the problems interfere with client functioning.

4. THIS PERSON HAS ABILITY TO COLLECT DATA AND IDENTIFY SIGNIFICANT CLIENT PROBLEMS. HE/SHE CAN SEE HOW THE PROBLEMS INTERFERE WITH CLIENT FUNCTIONING.

3. This person has some ability to collect data and identify client problems. He/she can see, to some extent, how the problems interfere with client functioning.
2. This person has deficiency collecting data and identifying client problems. He/she has difficulty appreciating how the problems interfere with client functioning.
1. This person is unable to collect data and identify client problems. He/she cannot see how the problems interfere with client functioning.

À LA CARTE DIMENSION N:

Identification of Alternative Courses of Clinical Disposition and Selection of an Intervention Plan

This dimension concerns your ability to design an intervention for a presenting problem. Can you identify different intervention possibilities? Can you see the implications for the client in these intervention options?

7. This person identifies a wide variety of alternative courses of clinical disposition, including those which may be creative and new, and reflective of extensive practice. The selection of an intervention plan is based on an experienced consideration of the consequences of the plan.

6. This person identifies a variety of alternative courses of clinical disposition, most of which have been applied successfully in similar situations. The selection of an intervention plan is based on an experienced consideration of the consequences of the plan.

5. This person can identify alternative courses of clinical disposition and select an appropriate intervention plan. The selection is also based upon a consideration of the consequences of the plan.

4. THIS PERSON CAN IDENTIFY ALTERNATIVE COURSES OF CLINICAL DISPOSITION AND CAN SELECT AN INTERVENTION PLAN.

3. This person has some capacity to identify alternative courses of disposition and has some ability to select an intervention plan. He/she does require assistance and supervision in this area.

2. This person has limited capability to identify alternative courses of clinical disposition and has difficulty selecting an intervention plan. He/she requires regular supervision in this area.

1. This person is unable to identify alternative courses of clinical disposition and cannot select an intervention plan.

À LA CARTE DIMENSION O:

Implementation and Evaluation of an Intervention Plan

This dimension examines your ability to apply an intervention. It also reflects your skills in evaluating the efficacy of your intervention with the client.

7. This person is superior in the implementation of an intervention plan. He/she expertly and effectively evaluates the intervention plan, and demonstrates a competence which reflects extensive experience and knowledge.
6. This person is remarkably skilful in the implementation of an intervention plan. He/she effectively evaluates the intervention plan, and demonstrates a competence which reflects experience and knowledge.
5. This person is skilful in the implementation of an intervention plan. He/she is effective in the evaluation of the plan.
4. THIS PERSON IS ABLE TO IMPLEMENT AN INTERVENTION PLAN. HE/SHE IS EFFECTIVE IN THE EVALUATION OF THE PLAN.
3. This person has some ability to implement an intervention plan. He/she can be effective in evaluating the plan. Support and supervision are occasionally required, however, in the administration of these skills.
2. This person has difficulty implementing an intervention plan. He/she has limitation in the evaluation of the plan. Consistent support and supervision are required in the administration of these skills.
1. This person is unable to implement an intervention plan. He/she is incapable of evaluating the plan.

À LA CARTE DIMENSION P:

Provision of an External Consultative Service

This dimension examines your knowledge base and skill level in the provision of external consultation. It is related only to your work environment, and does not examine the consultation process outside of this specific area. Can you do consultation where it is expected on your job, and can you consult with practicality and skill?

7. This person has a complete and thorough knowledge of the consultative process as it is applied in the work setting. He/she has a superior skill level, and provides consultation which demonstrates an appropriateness and practicality and is innovative when the situation merits.

6. This person has a complete knowledge of the consultative process as it is applied in the work setting. He/she has an extensive skill level, and provides consultation which demonstrates an appropriateness and practicality, and is innovative when the situation merits.

5. This person has a broad knowledge of the consultative process as it is applied in the work setting. He/she has an extensive skill level, and provides consultation which is appropriate and practical.

4. | THIS PERSON HAS KNOWLEDGE OF THE CONSULTATIVE PROCESS AS IT IS APPLIED IN THE WORK SETTING. HE/SHE HAS AN ACCEPTABLE SKILL LEVEL, AND PROVIDES CONSULTATION WHICH IS APPROPRIATE AND PRACTICAL.

3. This person has some knowledge of the consultative process as it is applied in the work setting. He/she approaches an acceptable skill level, and can provide consultation which is appropriate and practical.

2. This person has limited knowledge of the consultative process as it is applied in the work setting. He/she has difficulty achieving an acceptable skill level, and is inconsistent at the provision of consultation which is appropriate and practical.

1. This person has no knowledge of the consultation process as it is applied in the work setting. He/she is unable to achieve an acceptable skill level, and is incapable of providing consultation which is appropriate and practical.

À LA CARTE DIMENSION Q:

Ability to Demonstrate Oral and Written Communication Skills

This dimension asks you to evaluate your oral and written communication. Can you speak and write at an acceptable level for the expectations of your job? Do you need to work on these skills? This dimension is concerned only with oral and written aspects of work and does not consider additional aspects of these skills, which are reflected in other dimensions.

7. This person has superior oral and written communication skills. His/her communication displays remarkable clarity and quality and demonstrates an exquisite sensitivity to situations and events.
6. This person has excellent oral and written communication skills. His/her communication displays clarity and quality and demonstrates a sensitivity to situations and events.
5. This person is very competent in both oral and written communication skills. His/her communication shows both clarity and quality.
4. THIS PERSON IS COMPETENT IN BOTH ORAL AND WRITTEN COMMUNICATION SKILLS.
3. This person has some problems in oral or written communication and requires periodic instruction or supervision to improve the clarity or quality of these skills.
2. This person is limited in oral or written communication and requires regular instruction or supervision to improve the clarity or quality of these skills.
1. This person is not able to perform successfully in either oral or written communication. He/she does not have the skills to work efficiently in oral discussion, or lacks the basic skills of written communication.

À LA CARTE DIMENSION R:

Applied Knowledge of Child and Adolescent Care

This dimension is concerned with your knowledge of child and adolescent care and your ability to apply this knowledge. Do you require supervision to successfully apply your knowledge base? Is your knowledge base sufficient to allow you to work successfully with the target population?

7. This person has comprehensive knowledge of child and adolescent care. He/she can apply this knowledge successfully in practice, shows a realm of expertise in special situations, and serves as a resource person for others.
6. This person has thorough knowledge of child and adolescent care. He/she and can apply this knowledge successfully in practice, and with adaptability and a realm of expertise in special situations.
5. This person has full knowledge of child and adolescent care. He/she can apply this knowledge successfully in practice and shows adaptability to special situations.

4. THIS PERSON DEMONSTRATES KNOWLEDGE OF CHILD AND ADOLESCENT CARE. HE/SHE CAN APPLY THIS KNOWLEDGE SUCCESSFULLY IN PRACTICE.

3. This person has some knowledge of child and adolescent care and requires occasional instruction or supervision in the application of this knowledge.
2. This person has limited knowledge of child and adolescent care and requires regular instruction or supervision in the application of this knowledge.
1. This person does not have a knowledge of child and adolescent care and is unable to demonstrate any ability in the skills demanding the application of this knowledge.

À LA CARTE DIMENSION S:

Ability to Work as Part of a Team

This dimension examines your ability to work with other colleagues in a team situation. Can you integrate this demand into your individual performance? Do you integrate with the team in a supportive way? Do you work more individually and need to be reminded about teamwork?

7. This person vigorously and dynamically integrates teamwork and individual work. He/she continuously works collaboratively and skilfully with others, and is looked to for leadership in this regard.
6. This person vigorously integrates teamwork and individual work. He/she continuously works collaboratively with others in a supportive and skilful fashion.
5. This person actively integrates teamwork and individual work. He/she constantly works collaboratively with others in a supportive and skilful fashion.

4. THIS PERSON INTEGRATES TEAMWORK AND INDIVIDUAL WORK. HE/SHE WORKS COLLABORATIVELY WITH OTHERS IN A SUPPORTIVE AND SKILFUL FASHION.

3. This person attempts to integrate teamwork and individual work. He/she needs only periodic assistance or supervision to work collaboratively with others in a supportive and skilful fashion.
2. This person has difficulty integrating teamwork and individual work. He/she requires frequent reminders on these issues and requires assistance or supervision to work collaboratively with others in a supportive and skilful fashion.
1. This person is unsuccessful in teamwork and deliberately operates independently where teamwork is necessary. He/she fails to work collaboratively with others.

À LA CARTE DIMENSION T:

Management of Human Resources

This dimension asks you to consider some of the management aspects of your job. In the human management functions of recruiting others, or in supervision or evaluation, do you have the skills of communication, or information sharing, that are demanded? Do you understand group process as it applies to your personnel? Do you require some assistance in the provision of these functions, or are you meeting your performance expectations?

7. This person performs with excellence in functions involving staff recruitment, supervision and evaluation. He/she also shows confidence and self-assurance in the skills of communication, group process and information sharing. He/she can perform autonomously, shows adaptability and previous success in these management functions, and serves as a model for others in the provision of these skills.

6. This person performs with evident experience and expertise in functions involving staff recruitment, supervision, and evaluation. He/she also shows confidence and self-assurance in the skills of communication, group process and information sharing. He/she can perform autonomously and with proficiency, and shows an adaptability and range of skill reflective of previous success in these management functions.

5. This person performs with facility in functions involving staff recruitment, supervision and evaluation. He/she also shows confidence and self-assurance in the skills of communication, group process, and information sharing. He/she can function autonomously and with proficiency in the provision of these management functions.

4. | THIS PERSON PERFORMS COMPETENTLY IN THE MANAGEMENT FUNCTIONS OF STAFF RECRUIT-MENT, SUPERVISION, AND ON-GOING EVALUA-TION. HE/SHE HAS SKILLS IN COMMUNICATION, GROUP PROCESS, AND INFORMATION SHARING AND CAN FUNCTION AUTONOMOUSLY IN THE PROVISION OF THESE MANAGEMENT FUNC-TIONS.

3. This person can perform satisfactorily in functions involving staff recruitment, supervision, and evaluation and can show skills in communication, group process and information sharing. He/she does need periodic assistance or instruction in the provision of these functions.

2. This person is limited in some of the functions involving staff recruitment, supervision and evaluation and shows defeciency in communication, group process and information sharing. He/she requires regular and consistent reminders for the successful provision of these functions.

1. This person cannot perform satisfactorily in functions involving staff recruitment, supervision or evaluation and shows an absence of skills in communication, group process and information sharing.

À LA CARTE DIMENSION U:

Program Planning, Development and Evaluation

This dimension considers additional management functions. Can you deal with the program demands of your job? Are you able to design, implement and review program proposals? Can you collect information and delegate duties and responsibilities? Are you able to bring it all together so the program and personnel are integrated? Do you need assistance with these functions?

7. This person can expertly perform the skills of designing, implementing, and reviewing program proposals. He/she is proficient and resourceful in collecting and exchanging information with involved others, assigning roles and responsibilities, and integrating systems so that staff and programming work in concert. This is accomplished with efficiency and excellence, and shows a sensitivity to and appreciation of the individuals impacted through these functions.

6. This person can capably perform the skills of designing, implementing, and reviewing program proposals. He/she is proficient and resourceful in the essential aspects of collecting and exchanging information with involved others, assigning roles and responsibilities, and integrating systems so that staff and programming work in concert. This is accomplished with efficiency and excellence.

5. This person can capably perform the skills of designing, implementing and reviewing program proposals. He/she can also provide the essentials of collecting and exchanging information with involved others, assigning roles and responsibilities and integrating systems so that staff and programming work in concert. This is accomplished with evident efficiency and competence.

4.
THIS PERSON CAN PERFORM THE SKILLS OF DE-
SIGNING, IMPLEMENTING, AND REVIEWING
PROGRAM PROPOSALS. HE/SHE CAN ALSO PRO-
VIDE THE ESSENTIALS OF COLLECTING AND
EXCHANGING INFORMATION WITH INVOLVED
OTHERS, ASSIGNING ROLES AND RESPONSIBILI-
TIES, AND INTEGRATING SYSTEMS SO THAT
STAFF AND PROGRAMMING WORK IN CONCERT.

3. This person can satisfactorily perform some of the skills of designing, implementing, and reviewing program proposals. He/she can also provide some of the aspects of collecting and exchanging information with involved others, assigning roles and responsibilities, and integrating systems so that staff and programming work in concert. This is accomplished with periodic assistance or supervision.

2. This person has limitation in the skills of designing, implementing, and reviewing program proposals. He/she is also defecient in some aspects of collecting and exchanging information with involved others, assigning roles and responsibilities and integrating systems so that staff and programming work in concert. This is accomplished only with regular assistance and supervision.

1. This person cannot perform the skills of designing, implementing, and reviewing program proposals. He/she cannot provide the essential aspects of collecting and exchanging information with involved others, assigning roles and responsibilities, and integrating systems so that staff and programming work in concert.

À LA CARTE DIMENSION V:

Fiscal/Budget Planning and Management

This dimension looks at financial issues and budgetary demands. Are you able to prepare, monitor and review allocations? Are you able to consider personnel requests and demands in light of budgetary constraints? Can you collect and critically evaluate information about these aspects, or do you require assistance or supervision?

7. This person shows superior skill in the preparation, monitoring and reviewing of fiscal and budgetary allocations. He/she can sensitively examine and evaluate needs, and collect and critically consider fiscal or service requests. He/she demonstrates initiative and experience, and serves as a model for others in the performance of these skills.

6. This person shows excellence in the preparation, monitoring and reviewing of fiscal and budgetary allocations. He/she can sensitively examine and evaluate needs, collect and critically consider fiscal or service requests, and works with evident initiative and experience.

5. This person shows proficiency in the preparation, monitoring and reviewing of fiscal and budgetary allocations. He/she can sensitively examine and evaluate needs, and collect and critically consider fiscal or service requests.

4. THIS PERSON CAN PREPARE, MONITOR AND REVIEW FISCAL AND BUDGETARY ALLOCATIONS. HE/SHE CAN EXAMINE AND EVALUATE NEEDS, AND COLLECT AND CRITICALLY CONSIDER FISCAL OR SERVICE REQUESTS.

3. This person can sometimes prepare, monitor and review fiscal and budgetary allocations and can often examine and evaluate agency needs. He/she can collect and critically consider fiscal or service requests but requires periodic assistance or supervision.

2. This person is defecient in aspects of the preparation, monitoring or reviewing of fiscal and budgetary allocations and examining and evaluating agency needs. He/she can sometimes collect and critically consider fiscal or service requests but requires frequent and regular instruction or supervision.

1. This person is not able to successfully perform the functions of preparing, monitoring or reviewing fiscal or budgetary allocations, and cannot examine or evaluate agency needs. He/she is also unskilled in collecting or critically considering fiscal or service requests.

À LA CARTE DIMENSION W:

Agency Advocacy and Service Integration

This dimension examines your management skills at delivering the mandate and organizational plans of your service system. Are you able to promote and support their initiatives? Are you effective at relating between involved parties and personnel? Are you able to share goals, and have information flow through appropriate channels? Can you do this without assistance or supervision?

7. This person shows expertise in the development and recommendation of board service plans and objectives and sensitively promotes, supports and defends organizational interests and mandate. He/she demonstrates mastery of the interrelationships between affiliated boards and groups, and can smoothly arrange the flow and sharing of information among stakeholders.

6. This person shows excellence in the development and recommendation of board service plans and objectives and sensitively promotes, supports and defends organizational interests and mandate. He/she effectively and strategically interrelates between affiliated boards and groups and can arrange the flow and sharing of information among involved stakeholders.

5. This person appropriately develops and recommends board service plans and objectives, and promotes, supports and defends organizational interests and mandate. He/she effectively interrelates between affiliated boards and groups and arranges the flow and sharing of information among involved stakeholders.

4. THIS PERSON CAN DEVELOP AND RECOMMEND BOARD SERVICE PLANS AND OBJECTIVES, AND PROMOTE, SUPPORT AND DEFEND ORGANIZATIONAL INTERESTS AND MANDATE. HE/SHE CAN INTERRELATE BETWEEN AFFILIATED BOARDS AND GROUPS AND ARRANGES THE FLOW AND SHARING OF INFORMATION AMONG INVOLVED STAKEHOLDERS.

3. This person can sometimes develop and recommend board service plans and objectives, and can promote, support and defend organizational interests and mandate. He/she can often interrelate between affiliated boards and groups and arrange the flow and sharing of information among involved stakeholders but requires periodic assistance or instruction in these functions.

2. This person has limitation in the development and recommendation of board service plans and objectives, and has difficulty with some aspects of the promotion, support and defense of organizational interests and mandate. He/she attempts to interrelate between affiliated boards and groups and arrange the flow and sharing of information among involved stakeholders but requires frequent and regular instruction or supervision for the provision of these functions.

1. This person cannot develop and recommend board service plans and objectives and does not promote, support and defend organizational interests and mandate. He/she is unable to interrelate between affiliated boards and groups and does not arrange the flow and sharing of information among involved stakeholders.

À LA CARTE DIMENSION X:

Coordination of Client Services

This dimension examines your ability to coordinate activities in the delivery of integrated services to the client. You are asked to consider how well you communicate with others, mediate issues, set goals, and provide leadership in this aspect of client services.

7. This person can effectively and comfortably coordinate meetings, strategically negotiate with involved parties and set clear goals for expected service. He/she can sensitively mediate issues and provide a dynamic leadership function in the program. He/she serves as a model for others in the development of these skills.

6. This person can effectively and comfortably coordinate meetings, negotiate with involved parties, and set clear goals for expected service. He/she can sensitively mediate issues and provide an ongoing leadership function in the program.

5. This person can comfortably coordinate meetings, negotiate with involved parties, and set clear goals for expected service. He/she can also mediate issues and provide ongoing leadership functions in the program.

4. THIS PERSON CAN COORDINATE MEETINGS, NEGOTIATE WITH INVOLVED PARTIES, AND SET GOALS FOR EXPECTED SERVICE. HE/SHE CAN MEDIATE ISSUES AND PROVIDE AN ONGOING LEADERSHIP FUNCTION IN THE PROGRAM.

3. This person has some ability to coordinate meetings, negotiate with involved parties, and set goals for expected service. He/she also has some skills at mediating issues and providing an ongoing leadership function, but requires periodic assistance or supervision to successfully accomplish these job demands.

2. This person has limitations in the ability to coordinate meetings, negotiate with involved parties, and set goals for expected service. He/she also has difficulty mediating issues and providing ongoing leadership in the program. He/she requires continual assistance or supervision to successfully achieve the objectives.

1. This person does not have the ability to coordinate meetings, negotiate with involved parties and set goals for expected service. He/she is not able to mediate issues, or provide a leadership function.

À LA CARTE DIMENSION Y:

Ability to Demonstrate Office Practice Skills

This dimension considers the basic skills of office practice. Can you execute the expectations of your specific office job without assistance or supervision?

7. This person shows excellence in the execution of all aspects of office practice. He/she does so without assistance, works with evident experience, shows flexibility and a range of problem solving, and serves as a model for others in the execution of these skills.
6. This person shows proficiency in the execution of all aspects of office practice. He/she does so without assistance, works with evident experience, and shows a flexibility and range of problem solving reflective of extensive skill.
5. This person successfully executes the basic skills of office practice and does so without assistance, works comfortably, and with evident skill.

4. | THIS PERSON CAN SUCCESSFULLY EXECUTE THE BASIC SKILLS OF OFFICE PRACTICE. |

3. This person can successfully execute most of the basic skills of office practice but requires periodic instruction or supervision.
2. This person can successfully execute some of the basic skills of office practice and requires regular instruction and supervision.
1. This person cannot successfully execute the basic skills of office practice.

PERFORMANCE EVALUATION
INSTRUMENT SCORE SHEET

CORE DIMENSION A:
Establishment and Maintenance of Cooperative Relationships with
Colleagues

7   6   5   4   3   2   1

CORE DIMENSION B:
Understanding and Maintaining Relationships with Other Relevant
Organizations

7   6   5   4   3   2   1

CORE DIMENSION C:
Knowledge of the Characteristics of the Target Population

7   6   5   4   3   2   1

CORE DIMENSION D:
Awareness and Relevance of the Organization's Policies and Services to the Problems of the Target Population

7   6   5   4   3   2   1

CORE DIMENSION E:
Interpretation of the Organization to the Public

7   6   5   4   3   2   1

CORE DIMENSION F:
Knowledge and Use of Community Resources

7   6   5   4   3   2   1

CORE DIMENSION G:
Awareness and Commitment to Professional Values and Ethics

7   6   5   4   3   2   1

CORE DIMENSION H:
Responsibility for Individual Professional Development

7   6   5   4   3   2   1

CORE DIMENSION I:
Organization of Work and Time Management

7   6   5   4   3   2   1

CORE DIMENSION J:
Appropriate Use of Consultation and Supervision

7   6   5   4   3   2   1

CORE DIMENSION K:
Utilization and Provision of Organizationally Based Opportunities
for Staff Development

7   6   5   4   3   2   1

À LA CARTE DIMENSION L:
Establishment and Maintenance of a Professional Relationship with
Clients

7   6   5   4   3   2   1

À LA CARTE DIMENSION M:
Problem Identification and Assessment

7   6   5   4   3   2   1

À LA CARTE DIMENSION N:
Identification of Alternative Courses of Clinical Disposition and
Selection of an Intervention Plan

7   6   5   4   3   2   1

À LA CARTE DIMENSION O:
Implementation and Evaluation of An Intervention Plan

7   6   5   4   3   2   1

À LA CARTE DIMENSION P:
Provision of an External Consultative Service

7   6   5   4   3   2   1

À LA CARTE DIMENSION Q:
Ability to Demonstrate Oral and Written Communication Skills

7   6   5   4   3   2   1

À LA CARTE DIMENSION R:
Applied Knowledge of Child and Adolescent Care

| 7 | 6 | 5 | 4 | 3 | 2 | 1 |

À LA CARTE DIMENSION S:
Ability to Work as Part of a Team

| 7 | 6 | 5 | 4 | 3 | 2 | 1 |

À LA CARTE DIMENSION T:
Management of Human Resources

| 7 | 6 | 5 | 4 | 3 | 2 | 1 |

À LA CARTE DIMENSION U:
Program Planning, Development and Evaluation

| 7 | 6 | 5 | 4 | 3 | 2 | 1 |

À LA CARTE DIMENSION V:
Fiscal/Budget Planning and Management

| 7 | 6 | 5 | 4 | 3 | 2 | 1 |

À LA CARTE DIMENSION W:
Agency Advocacy and Service Integration

| 7 | 6 | 5 | 4 | 3 | 2 | 1 |

À LA CARTE DIMENSION X:
Coordination of Client Services

| 7 | 6 | 5 | 4 | 3 | 2 | 1 |

À LA CARTE DIMENSION Y:
Ability to Demonstrate Office Practice Skills

| 7 | 6 | 5 | 4 | 3 | 2 | 1 |

COMMENTS

STAFF MEMBER:

SUPERVISOR:

GOALS AND OBJECTIVES:

DATE

STAFF MEMBER

EXECUTIVE DIRECTOR

CLINICAL DIRECTOR

PROGRAM MANAGER

Chapter 6

Implementing the Process/
Using the Instrument

INTRODUCTION

Having the ideal performance evaluation instrument available for use in a human service organization is a necessary but insufficient condition for success. A process for using the instrument must be integrated into the organizational culture if the maximum benefits of the system are to be achieved. Operating alone, the tool is of little value if it simply sits on a shelf until the performance evaluation is due. Such an approach to evaluation does little to promote or support organizational standards. As well, it does not demonstrate a commitment to professional growth and development or a commitment to the employees and the work they do. What is required is a process whereby the instrument is introduced, constructed and then becomes a central component of organizational life. Together, the instrument and its process constitute a performance evaluation system. This chapter will describe this system.

"IDEAL" PERFORMANCE EVALUATION

The "ideal" performance evaluation instrument needs to be both comprehensive and, at the same time, uniquely responsive to the organization and the individuals involved. Both the instrument and the corresponding process must respect the fact that the organization and the employees within it have past experiences with evaluation, as well as their own standards and expectations of what should occur. In addition, the traps and pitfalls associated with "traditional" evaluation processes and instruments described in Chapter 1 must be avoided. This requires a carefully planned strategy which consists of four stages: (1) orientation of employees to the process and instrument; (2) time-frames for completion; (3) scoring procedures; and, (4) goal setting.

Orientation Phase

Implementation of the performance evaluation system needs to be preceded by an orientation to the instrument and process. As suggested in the previous chapter, this can be done through a general employee meeting or similar forum. As employees become active participants in the process of instrument development, various concerns can arise. In addition, assumptions and interpretations can form. Regular and continuous meetings during and after the development of the instrument can dispel these misperceptions.

Internal transfers from one program within an organization to another should also receive a re-orientation to the instrument through their new supervisor. The transfer may result in acquiring a new set of À LA CARTE dimensions and the transferred employee will now be evaluated on different components of the instrument. This demands a re-orientation to the tool and the process.

New employees should be briefed about the performance evaluation system during their orientation to employment with the agency. These employees bring with them their perceptions, attitudes, and personal recollections of previous performance appraisals. These need to be discussed at the time of orientation. This begins to foster in the new employee an appreciation and understanding of the ideology underlying the "ideal" instrument and process. Discussion with the new employee at this early stage also means that major tenets of the organizational culture, climate, philosophy, mission statement, and mandate can be articulated and reinforced. It also provides a chance for the employee to appreciate the congruence between the philosophy of the agency and the instrument and its process. The employee can come to a realization that the major principles that guide the organization can be translated into action through performance evaluation, and there can begin both a commitment to organizational standards and a genuine investment in professional growth and development.

Whether addressing new employees, existing employees, or staff transfers, the discussion of the performance evaluation instrument and process should not be delayed. Discussion about the philosophy and structure of the performance evaluation instrument is essential in avoiding difficulties that may arise in completing the instrument. The supervisor should review all the CORE and À LA CARTE dimensions concerned with the particular employee's job description. The employee should have a clear understanding of the instrument's structure and the scoring process. The User's Guide to the instrument can be helpful in augmenting this initial orientation to the performance evaluation system.

Time Frames

There are two major components to time frames. The first is concerned with the frequency of the performance evaluations–the intervals within which the performance evaluations are required through organizational policy. The second is the real time involved in the process of completing the performance evaluation.

Frequency

Typically, most organizations in the human service field place new employees on a six-month probationary period and then evaluate on a yearly basis thereafter. The first performance evaluation for new employees would, in that case, take place six months after beginning employment. Another evaluation should be done at the initial employment anniversary. Subsequently, staff should complete the performance evaluation once a year.

Real Time in the Process

The time involved in completing the performance evaluation instrument requires four steps. Initially, there is an orientation and familiarization with the instrument, usually associated with the orientation period with the organization. This is followed by the independent scoring by the employee and supervisor. Next comes a performance evaluation meeting to exchange and review scores and, finally, a meeting to identify goals for the coming year and to sign off.

Orientation time should be individualized and some employees may require more time than others. In most cases however, one can review and familiarize new staff about the key features of the system within one hour. This is, of course, a one-time event and is not repeated except in the case of an internal transfer.

The independent scoring involves approximately forty-five minutes by the employee and the supervisor. This activity is completed about two weeks before the face-to-face meeting. This meeting, at which both parties share their respective scores, should also take no more than an hour. The focus at this point is on sharing scores and addressing significant points of interest to both parties.

The final meeting occurs approximately two weeks after the one just described. The purpose of this meeting is to identify goals for the coming year. This engagement usually does not exceed half an hour.

Overall then, the total process can be accomplished in a four-hour period divided into four components. Since the orientation step is not repeated (except in the situation of an internal transfer), there are really only three steps, requiring about three hours, which form the basis for repeated evaluations. While each situation is unique and time can be collapsed or expanded as needed, three hours should serve as a general guideline for the more typical evaluation.

Scoring

The emphasis in the scoring should be on consistency in behavior across time. Both the worker and supervisor should guard against focusing on the most recent performance. They should also guard against focusing on any one specific incident. Attention needs to be paid to patterns of behavior or performance over time and not on critical incidents. With more senior employees, it is also important to remind them to confine the evaluation to the past year and not to performance in a previous year or to a cumulative evaluation of their entire career with the organization.

Face-to-Face Meeting

The face-to-face meeting has traditionally been the component of performance evaluation approached with the most trepidation by both supervisor and employee. However, using the performance evaluation instrument in the manner we have described can alleviate much of this difficulty since the independent scores on the instrument are the focal point for discussion. Both the employee and supervisor, having completed the instrument, have an idea of the major points they will want to address in their meeting. This meeting has two objectives: the sharing of scores and the addressing of areas of concern to either party.

Sharing the Scores

In the sharing of scores, the staff member should precede the supervisor. The reason for this is that the entire philosophy behind the process we advocate is violated if the supervisor leads, influences, or inadvertently suggests to the employee his/her perception of appropriate scores. We also recommend that the scores for all dimensions be reported completely before any significant dialogue occurs. This permits a global appreciation of the evaluation that comes from both sets of scores. It also avoids polarization or the risk of becoming focused on a single issue or on the first discrepant score. Chapter 7 provides more information and direction on addressing raw scores and patterns.

Content

The exchange of scores is an open process where neither the employee nor the supervisor is expected to provide an elaboration or clarification of their selections. During this part of the process, discrepancies in the scores between supervisor and employee will become apparent. A deviation of one, either higher or lower on the scale, should not be considered a significant discrepancy. A disparity of two or more, however, is significant, and should lead to discussion. Any discussion should wait until all the scores have been disclosed. The disparity in scores should be seen as opportunities to address specific issues and/or concerns. It is crucial that neither party become distracted by the range or variation in scores at this point. There may be a strong tendency or temptation to change the rating as a result of these observations. Neither the employee nor supervisor should be pressured or compelled to change their respective scores.

Scores Below the Benchmark

One of the most notable features of the instrument and process described here is the establishment of the benchmark. The benchmark is a neutral statement and is the expected or established standard of organizational performance. The supervisor will be concerned primarily with scores which fall below the benchmark since they convey failure to meet organizational expectations.

Since the supervisor has responsibility for ensuring that agency expectations are achieved and maintained, he/she will need to initiate discussion about these scores. This might occur, depending on the significance of a particular dimension to the agency, even if there was a discrepancy of only one between the score of the employee and that of the supervisor. Such discussion should focus first on whether there is confusion around the dimension. The discussion can then progress to whether the low score reflects a training issue, such as a lack of knowledge, information, or skill on the part of the employee.

The prevailing ambiance of this meeting should be a positive one where the focus is on education, training, and/or development. Furthermore, it should concentrate on bringing forward information to be shared between the employee and supervisor. The meeting should provide an opportunity to reach a clearer understanding and appreciation of where the individual and the organization are, and what they need to work toward. At the conclusion of the face-to-face meeting, the employee and supervisor schedule a follow-up meeting within two weeks to specifically discuss future goals.

Goal Setting

The final stage of the performance evaluation is the goal-setting stage. This part of the process should not require significant time if the substantial issues were identified in the previous face-to-face meeting. The goal-setting stage should concentrate on identifying mutual goals (usually three or four), to be accomplished before the next performance review. The employee should again initiate this discussion by identifying his/her goals. The supervisor's role is to determine if these match the administrative priorities of the performance evaluation. The supervisor may support, clarify or modify the goals, and/or include additional objective in discussion with the employee. Both parties can then include their respective comments on the evaluation form and sign off. This serves to indicate that both have read and reviewed the performance evaluation results.

Opportunity should be given to the employee at sign-off to record any disagreements he/she has with either the evaluation per se, or the goals set. Our experience, however, is that these disagreements are rare when the process is followed as we have described.

KEEPING THE PROCESS FRESH

One discovery we have made is that the requirement that supervisors or managers orient new and transferred employees to the instrument and process, serves to keep it current and "fresh." During the course of such an orientation, it can occur to the manager that certain dimensions, or the wording of the dimensions, have not stood the test of time. Changes may have been required as the organization expanded, contracted, or altered its mission or goals. This "jogging of awareness" is a healthy process because no "ideal" process or instrument can stay that way indefinitely. The ideal instrument must be adapted to fit new or different realities in order to keep it "ideal."

Even with this kind of informal, continual review, we recommend, as standard practice, a formal review process every few years. At this time, the process and instrument should become the focus of a staff meeting. The manager should take this agenda item seriously and ask employees to review the content and procedures with vigor. This review is intended to identify changes that may be required to keep the process and instrument "fresh" and to promote staff involvement with, and acceptance of, these changes.

Chapter 7

The "Ideal" Performance System in Action

In the face-to-face meeting the parties come together to review their individual scores, and to talk about the implications of these scores for the future. When the scores are identified–initially by the employee and then by the supervisor–various patterns and profiles will become evident. The scoring profiles will indicate either considerable agreement or evident disagreement between supervisor and employee. These similarities and differences need to be handled differently. We recommend two particular methods to examine individual score profiles: the "Synoptic" and "Focused" reviews.

As a further point to consider in the handling of the scoring profiles, remember that the profiles and their patterns are about individual employees. However, most people operate within a job group. Other employees are doing the same job and hence, will be considered on the same dimensions. This means that for purposes of analyzing a total program, or looking critically at a complete job group, all the individual scores could be aggregated. This compilation of scores could provide the profile or pattern of scores presented by the entire staff in an identified program. A composite evaluation of a complete job group is called the "Systemic" method of review.

The instrument and process can therefore accommodate three different approaches to the utilization of evaluation results. The first two, Synoptic and Focused, are specifically oriented to an evaluation of an individual employee. The Systemic method is particularly useful in evaluating the entire organization or any program within the organization.

APPLYING THE SYNOPTIC AND FOCUSED METHODS

The examples provided in this section are profiles that were identified through the use of the "ideal" performance evaluation instrument in a children's mental health agency with a variety of programs and services. Individual profiles are considered initially and will reveal significant information about specific issues and patterns that emerge in the unique job functions when viewed by both the employee and supervisor.

THE SYNOPTIC METHOD

The Synoptic method is utilized when there is a high correlation in the scores between employee and supervisor and there are no disparities greater than one. The disclosure of scores is initiated by the employee who provides a complete presentation of his/her scores on all dimensions. This is followed by the supervisor sharing his/her scores. The discussion is open-ended and the participants utilize the synopsis of the scores as the opportunity to provide feedback, to reinforce certain areas, to attend to those issues which may still demand some dialogue, and to address career and training interests. The intention is to provide sufficient time for any required interaction, and to identify and capitalize on the "kernels of substance" that are revealed in the relationship of the scores to each other. Figure 1 illustrates a profile where at first glance there appears to be considerable agreement and the Synoptic method of review is recommended.

The scores in this example present an interesting pattern because of the high degree of consensus between employee and supervisor. Initially there does not seem to be a great deal to discuss, other than to mutually agree, and there may be a strong temptation to terminate the meeting quickly. However, the supervisor and employee may both be making an assumption that, if followed, could result in a lost opportunity to address issues that are relevant and important. Despite the high degree of consensus, there is not a perfect correlation in the profile. A quick scan of the results indicates that there are small points of disagreement and, indeed, on one dimension the

FIGURE 1

Dimensions	Scores	
	Employee	**Supervisor**
CORE DIM. A	5	5
CORE DIM. B	4	3
CORE DIM. C	5	6
CORE DIM. D	6	5
CORE DIM. E	5	6
CORE DIM. F	4	5
CORE DIM. G	6	6
CORE DIM. H	4	5
CORE DIM. I	5	5
CORE DIM. J	5	5
CORE DIM. K	4	5
À LA CARTE L	4	5
À LA CARTE M	5	6
À LA CARTE N	5	5
À LA CARTE O	6	5
À LA CARTE Q	6	6

supervisor has rated the employee below the benchmark (CORE Dimension B).

The interaction between supervisor and employee should focus on those particular dimensions involving disagreement and should result in clarification and understanding about the behaviors that led to these scores. A further glance at the profile reveals that the majority of scores are higher than the benchmark. It is important that both parties discuss this point. From this observation, useful discussion about further professional growth opportunities, career advancements, and so forth, can ensue.

We emphasize that this type of profile demands a particular form of review. The supervisor needs to focus on certain important features. Are there any scores below the benchmark? Who gave those ratings–supervisor, employee, or both? Are there scores much higher than the benchmark? Who determined these? Did both people agree on the key dimensions or are the differences only one point on the scale? These features are some of the significant considerations in a Synoptic profile.

THE FOCUSED METHOD

The second method available to address the scoring at the face-to-face meeting is the Focused approach. The Focused review requires that the evaluators address any blatant disparities first. These are dimensions where there are significant differences in scores. Figure 2 provides a scoring profile which demands the utilization of the Focused method. The profile clearly reflects some differences of opinion between supervisor and employee.

As can be seen, there are differences of greater than one between supervisor and employee on CORE Dimension J and À LA CARTE Dimension O. The Focused method requires that initial attention be paid to these scores. It is possible that the entire review will be taken up with a discussion of these scores. If this occurs, it should not raise any unnecessary concern. It may very well be that this is *the* content critical to the performance evaluation process. Consequently, little opportunity may exist to search for, and address, the material which forms the basis for a Synoptic evaluation. If time remains, there is virtue in applying the Synoptic approach to the

FIGURE 2

Dimensions	Scores	
	Employee	Supervisor
CORE DIM. A	5	5
CORE DIM. B	6	6
CORE DIM. C	6	6
CORE DIM. D	5	5
CORE DIM. E	5	4
CORE DIM. F	5	5
CORE DIM. G	5	5
CORE DIM. H	6	5
CORE DIM. I	5	5
CORE DIM. J	6	4
CORE DIM. K	6	6
À LA CARTE L	5	5
À LA CARTE M	5	5
À LA CARTE N	5	4
À LA CARTE O	5	3
À LA CARTE Q	5	5

remaining scores. The opportunity should obviously not be lost to find positive and constructive items to discuss and compare. It should be emphasized that the theme of both methods is the future. To ignore this central point is to court disagreement, and potentiate an unpleasant atmosphere.

THE SYSTEMIC METHOD

One of the most attractive features of the "ideal" performance evaluation scoring format represented in this text is that it has the capacity to provide a Systemic overview of the entire organization, or a particular job group within that organization. This is easily accomplished by aggregating the results of all the performance scores of each member of the job group over a particular time period, and then rounding off a mean score to the nearest whole number.

In Figure 3 that follows, the scores of a group of employees working with emotionally disturbed children in the residential program of a children's mental health agency are illustrated. All workers have completed the same dimensions and the same supervisor has been a party to each evaluation. By establishing the mean score of the employees on each dimension, a group profile can be plotted. The supervisor's scores on each dimension are then plotted on the group profile. What becomes available is a Systemic overview of a program's scores across a particular time period.

This information can be extremely valuable for the organization. In fact, the major benefits of this data are toward organizational objectives. Implications for staff development and training, future human resource planning, and concerns regarding strengths and weaknesses in the existing organizational programs or structures, could result from a review of this data.

The evaluation of this profile should be approached in the same manner as one would with an individual and rely again on either the Synoptic or Focused method. However, in this instance the supervisor is the only party to the process.

In the example, there are dimensions which suggest the Focused approach as the initial step (CORE Dimension C). Since discussion is not required–indeed not even possible unless you collect all

FIGURE 3

Dimensions	Scores	
	Employees	Supervisor
CORE DIM. A	4	4
CORE DIM. B	4	4
CORE DIM. C	3	5
CORE DIM. D	4	5
CORE DIM. E	4	5
CORE DIM. F	5	5
CORE DIM. G	6	6
CORE DIM. H	5	4
CORE DIM. I	5	5
CORE DIM. J	5	4
CORE DIM. K	4	4
À LA CARTE L	6	5
À LA CARTE M	5	4
À LA CARTE Q	5	4
À LA CARTE R	5	5
À LA CARTE S	5	5

NOTE: All mean scores have been rounded to the nearest whole number.

members of the job group together–the information from the discrepant scores is gleaned from the supervisor's own appreciation of the meaning of the data. This is not time consuming and opportunity exists to return to a Synoptic appreciation of the profile. Both approaches can and should be used in the Systemic evaluation.

Information provided through the Systemic evaluation can be used in several ways. Initially, the supervisor can try to address his/her discoveries by making unilateral program changes or adaptations. It may not be necessary to involve the participating players in this decision. However, there will be occasions when the information is so important, or the suggested changes indicate such delicate human resource consequences, that it requires a group meeting. The supervisor could then engage the work group in problem solving or use the meeting as a medium to address the discoveries.

The Systemic evaluation can have broader applicability. For example, it can serve as the basis for managerial level discussions. From such discussions can develop ideas and plans concerning future directions for the organization, human resource management, recruitment, and training opportunities.

Earlier, we noted the importance of regular and systematic audit of the instrument in order to keep it viable and current. At the time we stressed the use of the employee-supervisor meeting to accomplish this end. The Systemic method also provides an opportunity to evaluate the utility of the performance evaluation instrument and can serve as a quality control mechanism to measure its practicality and efficacy. Changes in the organization over time, and the ability of the tool to respond to these changes, will become apparent in the appropriateness of the instrument at this stage in the development of the organization. Changes and adaptations may have to be made to the performance evaluation instrument to make it "ideal" again. The Systemic method is one way of addressing this organizational responsibility.

THE SYNOPTIC AND FOCUSED METHODS IN ACTION

In order to enhance the reader's appreciation of the performance evaluation instrument in action, we will present four very common individual profiles and look at how the performance review, based on the scores, should be conducted. The profiles are those of a new employee, a senior employee, a manager/supervisor, and last, but certainly not least, a problematic employee.

These examples were chosen because they represent a broad cross-section of the kinds of employees frequently found in most human service organizations. The examples are authentic and the scores are those actually provided by both the employee and the supervisor. In three of the cases, there are two supervisors involved, and this is explained through the discussion of the results. Following the four individual profiles, we will provide an example of the Systemic method in action through a clinical team review.

The New Employee

The new employee commonly presents a profile where the scores are modest and congregate near the benchmark. It is not unusual to find that there are no discrepancies greater than one and, if there are, they are few in number. In this example of an evaluation of a new employee (Figure 4), it can be noted that there is one dimension where there is a two-point discrepancy (CORE Dimension E), but the discrepancy is on the scoring of a single supervisor and is not shared by the co-supervisor.

With new employees, the evaluation frequently occurs on the sixth-month anniversary date. This is considered the probationary period and, as a result, the parties are operating with fairly limited information. This may contribute to the clustering of the scores near the benchmark. Another is the fact that some new employees are in their first professional job.

Profiles of new employees typically reveal more concerns (i.e., low scores) on the À LA CARTE Dimensions than the CORE Dimensions. The CORE Dimensions deal with behaviors which are, for the most part, generic to human service work. New employees normally bring these skills with them as a consequence of previous experience and/or professional education and training. On the other hand, the À LA CARTE Dimensions measure skills specific to a

FIGURE 4: THE NEW EMPLOYEE

Dimensions	Scores		
	Employee	Supervisor	Clinical Director
CORE DIM. A	4	4	4
CORE DIM. B	5	4	4
CORE DIM. C	4	4	5
CORE DIM. D	5	5	4
CORE DIM. E	5	3	4
CORE DIM. F	3	4	3
CORE DIM. G	4	4	5
CORE DIM. H	4	4	4
CORE DIM. I	5	4	4
CORE DIM. J	4	5	4
CORE DIM. K	5	5	4
À LA CARTE L	4	4	3
À LA CARTE M	5	4	4
À LA CARTE N	4	3	3
À LA CARTE O	4	4	4

particular job. It is understandable that these skills might be performed at a lower level during the first few months of employment.

Figure 4 illustrates scores from an employee and his/her two supervisors. In this particular case, the employee has both administrative and clinical functions and, as a consequence, reports to two people. The scores show that, for the most part, performance is in line with expectations. The scores are at the benchmark on the majority of dimensions although there are some minor issues that should be addressed.

Following a Focused approach, the review should begin with a discussion about Dimension E, the only scale on which there is a difference of greater than one between evaluators. Most certainly, the supervisors will also want to discuss Dimensions F, L, and N with the employee since in the view of at least one of them, performance was below the benchmark on these dimensions.

A Synoptic review could then be used to address other issues. In the example given it can be seen that the employee tends to rate himself/herself slightly higher than either supervisor. A fruitful discussion could occur around this point that could lead to a better understanding of supervisory expectations as well as defuse any resentment or bad feelings on the part of the employee that his/her supervisor(s) has(have) been too harsh.

The profile of this probationary employee is typical of that seen for this group of employees. The employee tends to be modest in the portrayal of his/her abilities and the scores of the supervisor indicate a basic satisfaction with the performance to date along with some areas "flagged" for discussion and improvement. As noted previously, shortcomings are more typically seen in the À LA CARTE Dimensions pertaining to specific behaviors relating to a particular job. One finds that as employees continue in a job, attention will shift to broader areas pertaining to agency mission, generic professional behavior and so forth. In other words, CORE Dimensions become more important areas of attention and concentration as the employee remains with the organization.

The Senior Employee

The profile of this senior employee (Figure 5) shows a pattern of scores which exceed the benchmark. This is not unusual and, in

FIGURE 5: THE SENIOR EMPLOYEE

Dimensions	Scores		
	Employee	Supervisor	Clinical Director
CORE DIM. A	6	6	6
CORE DIM. B	6	5	6
CORE DIM. C	5	5	5
CORE DIM. D	6	4	4
CORE DIM. E	5	6	6
CORE DIM. F	6	5	6
CORE DIM. G	6	6	6
CORE DIM. H	6	6	5
CORE DIM. I	5	3	4
CORE DIM. J	6	4	5
CORE DIM. K	5	5	5
À LA CARTE L	6	5	5
À LA CARTE M	5	5	5
À LA CARTE N	5	4	5
À LA CARTE O	5	6	6
À LA CARTE Q	4	4	5
À LA CARTE R	4	4	4
À LA CARTE S	5	5	5

fact, one would hope that this would be the case. The profile suggests beginning with the Focused method of review, concentrating on CORE Dimensions D, I, and J, the three dimensions with differences between employee and supervisor(s) of greater than one.

One observes in this profile that the differences between supervisor(s) and employee are all on CORE Dimensions. This is frequently the case with the senior employee. Our experience is that when employees are retained in an organization for long periods of time, issues concerning specific skills related to a particular task or job cease to be a major focus of the annual evaluation. This is not to devalue the À LA CARTE Dimensions as an important focus for senior employees because performance can deteriorate and this can be picked up by the instrument. There are also professional development issues in the À LA CARTE Dimensions that need discussing. Nevertheless, the major focus of the performance review is generally on broader issues relating to agency policies, procedures, and mandate, as well as overall professional comportment.

In the example provided, a Focused approach would concentrate on Dimensions D, I, and J. This should be followed by a Synoptic review of the complete picture presented by the scores. When senior staff members are being evaluated, the Synoptic method of review should not be overlooked because there are professional development issues that are paramount for these individuals. The development issues are not the same for senior staff as they are for new employees because basic skill levels have often been attained and professional development and personal expertise is now at the forefront. Normally, one does not find much discrepancy between evaluator and evaluatee scores on the À LA CARTE Dimensions. This congruency can cause the professional goal-setting component of the process to be overlooked because attention was riveted on the disparities noted on the CORE Dimensions. The use of the Synoptic review allows the evaluation to return to more congenial issues relating to professional development and moves it to a focus on the future.

The Program Manager

The management-level employee (Figure 6) is evaluated on the same CORE Dimensions as all other personnel. The differences in the evaluation dimensions exist only on the À LA CARTE Dimensions where the management individuals will address dimensions relating to such tasks as program planning, budget control, supervision of personnel, and teamwork.

Evaluating management-level personnel on the same CORE Dimensions as all other personnel is an attractive feature of the "ideal" performance evaluation instrument. A philosophy of egalitarianism is actualized through this process and is consistent with the "one size fits all" concept discussed earlier.

In the example provided the scores are quite close and tend to cluster around the baseline, or slightly above. A composite profile of the scores seems to indicate that both parties feel very comfortable with the current situation and there are no outstanding issues. There are no scores below the benchmark by either party so there is no evidence that, from an organizational perspective, a problem exists which would require any immediate training or supervision.

Given the high congruency in scores there is a temptation to adjourn the evaluation session quickly. We believe this would be

FIGURE 6: PROGRAM MANAGER

Dimensions	Scores	
	Program Manager	Administrator
CORE DIM. A	5	4
CORE DIM. B	4	5
CORE DIM. C	5	5
CORE DIM. D	5	6
CORE DIM. E	5	4
CORE DIM. F	5	6
CORE DIM. G	5	5
CORE DIM. H	5	6
CORE DIM. I	5	5
CORE DIM. J	5	4
CORE DIM. K	4	5
À LA CARTE Q	4	5
À LA CARTE S	4	4
À LA CARTE T	4	5
À LA CARTE U	4	5
À LA CARTE V	4	4

premature. We recommend instead that the Synoptic method be employed. There is material here which suggests that there are things to discuss, and there is an opportunity to provide some positive reinforcement to the program manager when the total picture seems to indicate that things are operating in a promising fashion.

The Problematic Employee

Despite the appearance of a "manufactured" profile to amplify the dramatic differences between the supervisors' and employee's scores, Figure 7 represents an actual situation encountered by two of the authors. Quite clearly, the employee has a very different image of his/her abilities than the supervisor and the clinical director. As one can observe, the employee does not feel there is even one identifiable problem. The scores given by the staff member, in contrast to the supervisors, indicate that he/she believes that his/her performance exceeds the benchmark on every dimension, and reaches the highest professional standard (7) on five of the dimensions.

FIGURE 7: THE PROBLEMATIC EMPLOYEE

Dimensions	Employee	Supervisor	Clinical Director
		Scores	
CORE DIM. A	5	3	4
CORE DIM. B	4	4	4
CORE DIM. C	5	3	3
CORE DIM. D	6	4	3
CORE DIM. E	6	4	4
CORE DIM. F	6	4	4
CORE DIM. G	7	4	4
CORE DIM. H	7	3	3
CORE DIM. I	5	2	3
CORE DIM. J	7	3	3
CORE DIM. K	7	2	3
À LA CARTE L	7	3	3
À LA CARTE N	6	3	3
À LA CARTE Q	6	4	4
À LA CARTE R	6	2	3
À LA CARTE S	6	2	2

Our experience with the "ideal" performance evaluation instrument leads us to assert that this particular pattern of exaggerated self-scoring is a "marker" for problematic employees. Such an employee tends to deny the issues and, indeed, will argue that he/she has very little idea what the supervisor is talking about. These staff members can present a remarkable amount of rigidity in the face of the obvious differences in opinion between them and their supervisors. An obvious problem is that the employee in our example seems to have no sense of perspective. As can be seen, he/she provides scores which border on perfection.

The choice of evaluation method to use in this profile seems obvious at the outset since there are so many discrepancies. The recommended method is the Focused approach. In the case of the problematic employee this presents a dilemma because it is not clear where to start. In our example, there are 15 differences greater than one for the supervisor, and 14 differences greater than one for the clinical director. One of these differences is as great as five (5)! The Focused approach should still be attempted as a starting point and a beginning could be made with the dimension which has the most glaring differences. In the example, this would be CORE Dimension K.

What happens from this point is dependent upon both the employee's willingness to engage in constructive dialogue about his/her deficiencies in performance and the position taken by management about the future status of this employee. We have emphasized that the functions and purposes of performance evaluation are toward professional development and aimed at the future of the employee. This is not a position that naively fails to recognize that individuals can have serious problems that adversely effect their professional performance. Similarly, there are employees who are clearly working in a job that is not suited to their skills or their particular character.

Obviously, decisions must be made about the possibility of retention of such an employee. Our experience has been that transferring such a staff member does not resolve the situation if the problems are based in the personality of the actor. It is an unfortunate fact that some employees cannot be retained when these realities become apparent. The "ideal" performance evaluation makes these very difficult decisions less stressful because the differences are quantifiable and apparent and are not based on vague, subjective data.

THE SYSTEMIC METHOD IN ACTION: A CLINICAL TEAM REVIEW

The results shown in Figure 8 are the aggregate scores for the members of a clinical team that delivers outpatient therapeutic service to children and families. The scores have been averaged and then rounded to the nearest whole number.

The team is administered by a program manager and receives clinical supervision from the clinical director of the children's agency. There are 11 staff being considered. All the evaluations involved both the program manager and the clinical director since they shared responsibilities for the supervision and for the annual reviews.

In the systemic evaluation, the information is relevant for the administration of the agency and most specifically for the two supervisors directly involved with these professionals. The scores can

FIGURE 8: CLINICAL TEAM REVIEW
USING THE SYSTEMIC APPROACH

Dimensions	Scores		
	Clinicians	Program Manager	Clinical Director
CORE DIM. A	4	4	4
CORE DIM. B	4	4	5
CORE DIM. C	4	4	4
CORE DIM. D	4	5	5
CORE DIM. E	5	5	5
CORE DIM. F	5	5	4
CORE DIM. G	6	6	5
CORE DIM. H	4	4	5
CORE DIM. I	5	5	5
CORE DIM. J	5	4	4
CORE DIM. K	4	5	4
À LA CARTE L	5	4	4
À LA CARTE M	5	4	4
À LA CARTE N	6	4	5
À LA CARTE O	4	4	4
À LA CARTE Q	5	4	4
À LA CARTE R	5	5	5
À LA CARTE S	5	5	5

reveal the strengths and weaknesses of the program. The purpose is not to isolate individuals–and it is impossible to do so unless you were to return to the original documents–but to get a comprehensive overview of the way the program is viewed by the staff and the supervisors, and to see whether both groups are really operating within the same frame of reference. There may be occasions when one of the individual evaluations should be discarded–as with the problematic employee whose scores may be so distorted that they are not representative of the program.

The systemic evaluation is treated exactly the same as a review of an individual. It should be looked at from both a focused and synoptic approach. In this case, where there are two supervisors, it can be an opportunity for dialogue about the scores. In most cases, there is only a single supervisor and the systemic review provides little occasion for conversation and more for personal reflection. It is always possible to return to the team with the results if interaction or clarity around the results is the goal. Indeed, this provides a healthy occasion for program evaluation involving all staff. Among other things, it demonstrates an openness of management toward staff feedback and input and represents a responsiveness to staff that is quite progressive.

If we consider this systemic review from the focused approach, there is only one dimension (À LA CARTE N) which shows a disparity greater than one. The program manager has rated the staff at the benchmark (4) and the staff have scored themselves at 6. The clinical director has averaged 5 for the staff on this dimension. The dimension is entitled "Clinical Disposition and Development of an Intervention Plan."

The discrepancy in scores can initiate discussion in a number of interesting ways. Since the clinical director and staff are within one point of each other and would, seemingly, have a deeper understanding of the operational side of this dimension, does the program manager have a complete grasp of the clinical aspects? Or, are the staff over-scoring their skill level as a group since both the program manager and clinical director have scores that are below the staff average by at least a full point?

This could form the substance of dialogue between the two supervisors and a plan to address their conclusions could be put into place. It might involve clarifying various aspects of the dimension for the program manager's benefit and, as a result, he/she would be able to more accurately evaluate this dimension in subsequent reviews. Or it might lead to the conclusion that the staff need to meet with the supervisors to review this finding and explore the reasons for the apparent differences of opinion.

The systemic evaluation can now move to a synoptic examination of the remaining dimensions. In this case there are ten dimensions which show a difference of one (1) and seven (7) that are a perfect match. The first thing to appreciate is that the staff and supervisors are in considerable agreement about the program. Since none of the scores are below the baseline, it can also be comforting to know that people feel competent about the job they are doing, and the supervisors generally concur with this self-evaluation.

Chapter 8

The Ideal Performance Evaluation System: Applications and Implications

Any attempt at designing, implementing, and conducting a new approach to performance evaluation should be expected to have problems, and this one is not exceptional. However, we believe the advantages and assets of the system far outweigh its limitations. In this closing chapter, the strengths and weaknesses of the system are highlighted and suggestions are offered for its further development. In so doing, the evaluation system is discussed from three different perspectives: the staff, administration/management, and the organization as a whole.

STAFF CONSIDERATIONS IN THE IDEAL SYSTEM

The major strength of the system, from a staff perspective, is that it is responsive to them. The ideal system meets its promise of being consumer-responsive. The results of meeting this goal are found in improved communication between staff and management, and heightened motivation in the workplace.

Our experience is that it is more frequently *the worker* who initiates a reminder that the performance evaluation review date is forthcoming. Furthermore, since the evaluation results are not associated with pay or bonuses, his/her motivation for this reminder is more clearly related to the process itself and not toward an anticipated financial outcome.

This leads us to the belief that there is greater trust in the system of evaluation. The opportunity to participate in the development of the dimensions, the involvement in both building the dimensions and in clarifying the language of the scales, seem to have lessened the suspicion usually associated with evaluation as an administratively driven process.

There is also a genuine sense of team involvement in the collaboration and co-determination of a product which has real impact on all the players. The evaluation system has moved away from a foreign tool which is imposed on participants to a familiar instrument which contains no surprises. The skepticism has been reduced or eliminated and there is an assurance that the evaluation process is just and fair.

This element of fairness is increased by the knowledge that the same system of evaluation is being used for management. Since the CORE dimensions are universal and only the À LA CARTE dimensions are unique to the job groups, this awareness of universality of dimensions, as well as the knowledge that there is a commitment to the same process of application of the instrument, contributes to a sense of egalitarianism.

One noticeable outcome of the development of the ideal system has been that the building of À LA CARTE dimensions in a collaborative fashion has removed some of the air of mystery and mystique which pervades clinical work. The clinical providers in human service have had to describe and define more clearly what it is they are doing when they are involved in therapy, or the business of change. This has not been an easy task but it has led to the description of service roles which are, to some extent at least, more objective, concrete, and measurable.

The cost to workers, however, has been that they have had to let go of the belief that what they do defies description and quantification and is therefore indeterminate by anyone outside of its actual practice. It was easier for them to reject evaluation systems which were built by others, or borrowed from other systems, because they could, in a sense, take shelter behind this thinking.

Another discovery in the utilization of the ideal system has been that staff are more comfortable with the "agree to disagree" option of the scoring system. In the ideal system the participants do not have to change their scores. They just agree to leave things as they are if the parties cannot see each other's point of view.

Perhaps the sense of comfort with the "agree to disagree" component of the process for staff coincides with the perception that the ideal evaluation has reduced the reward power of the supervisor. In the traditional appraisal system, the supervisor is in a hierarchical position by virtue of the fact that the ratings were often determined solely by him/her, and these scores could potentially determine the pay increase, promotion opportunities, and even one's future with the organization. In the ideal system, there is no demand for consensus and the worker's ratings are considered to be just as credible as those of the supervisor.

Of course, the downside of this philosophy of "agree to disagree" is that it can be a two-edged sword. The supervisor, like the staff member, is under no obligation to change his/her ratings. Hence, the potential exists for a permanent record of a low rating. However, since in most appraisal systems there is far more pressure on the staff member to bring his/her scores in line with those of the supervisor than vice versa, this problem (from the employee's perspective) may be more imagined than real.

We have found that the collaboration of workers and supervisors/administrators in the construction of the system leads to the development of a deeper level of appreciation in the direct service staff of the functions and purposes of the supervisory/administrative system. The staff are able to see the "big picture" of service as a blend of sound management and superior service provision, and they become more appreciative of the concerns and constraints of supervision/administration.

Staff also find that there is more to the agency than the limited interests directly connected to their particular service role, and they realize that the agency has larger expectations for the employee. These are explicitly expressed in the CORE dimensions–issues such as the agency's mission and mandate–and the relevance of agency policy to these spheres. The presence of fundamental organizational concerns, reflected through the CORE dimensions, and the fact that staff are involved in their development and language, all serve to assist in moving the provider group toward a stronger sense of respect for the supervisory/administrative aspects of the service system.

As a final consideration of the impact of the ideal evaluation system on staff, our experience shows that workers are very attracted to the ability of the system to separate the evaluative/judgmental aspects of the evaluation from the educational/developmental aspects. The reader will recall that this is accomplished by the benchmark which serves to establish the administrative ceiling at step four on the dimension and leaves the last three steps for professional growth and development. This is considered a positive contribution of the system and a clear and evident demonstration of agency responsiveness to its staff.

A danger that staff and management must guard against is complacency with the system. A reduction in anxiety about performance evaluation can be accompanied by a "if it ain't broke, don't fix it" mind-set. This is compounded by the fact that scale building is not easy work. It is important to emphasize that the ideal system needs regular maintenance and overhaul and updating and managing the system can become a joint partnership of staff and management.

SUPERVISOR/ADMINISTRATIVE CONSIDERATIONS IN THE IDEAL SYSTEM

Earlier, we noted that engaging direct service personnel in the specification of their job duties removed some of the clinical mystique. We alluded to the fact that, to a certain extent, this constituted a certain loss of power for the worker vis-à-vis his/her supervisor. Since the client-worker relationship occurs outside the direct purview of the supervisor, the worker can, in effect, engage in some "broken field running" when it comes to the evaluation of direct service areas. When the evaluation instruments are built by managers, or borrowed from other systems, workers can claim that their work is too abstract and subjective to be evaluated. Or they might argue that this area can only be understood by fellow clinicians who are able to appreciate the subtlety of their work.

In this fashion, the evaluation of intervention strategies and techniques, use of theory, responsiveness to clients, and so forth is avoided. Instead, the evaluation is kept on a more administrative level such as number of cases opened, closed, or maintained, time management, and case recording issues.

The ideal system opens up this area for description and subsequently for scrutiny and evaluation. The supervisor/administrator can now participate in the adjudication of those areas previously defined as sacred by the service provider and considered as resistant to description and review. This eliminates a subtle power disparity that was described a number of years ago in a humorous fashion by Alfred Kadushin (1968).

In the previous section, we noted that the "agree to disagree" concept, while having some real advantages to workers, was also a two-edged sword. By always having two evaluations on record (the worker's and the supervisor's), disparate ratings are accentuated and differences between worker and management are readily apparent. Hence, a "paper trail" begins to develop which may be required in future disciplinary actions or termination.

Our intent throughout this book has been to emphasize a system that is focused on helping staff members come to an honest appraisal of their competency. We are also deeply committed to the belief that people have the capacity to grow and change. However, we are not so naive to believe that a loyalty to this philosophy always leads to a good result. The ideal system also provides management with the information needed to support serious corrective action.

One feature of the ideal system which is an additional asset to supervision/administration is that the evaluative system can become a venue for issues which are sensitive or controversial. Because it is so comprehensive and all-inclusive, it is possible to find an opportunity to address concerns which might not find a forum. The behavior of colleagues toward one another is an example, or where a worker is observed becoming too familiar with his/her clients. In more traditional appraisal systems, such issues can be easily avoided. This can lead to future embarrassment for the staff member and the agency. It can also mean that when it does become too big to hide, it can lead to charges of unfair dismissal and possible litigation.

We emphasize again that the ideal system encourages a particular ideology and attitude about evaluation and demands that the supervisor/administrator accept that philosophy. It requires management to let go of traditional hierarchical notions about appraisal and move instead toward a partnership with staff in the design and construction of the evaluation system. Clearly, this can arouse resistance on the part of management who fear a loss of control.

For those supervisors/administrators who are able to make the successful transition from the hierarchical model to this responsive approach, a discovery is made that evaluation is not something that is a chore and an unpleasant requirement of the job. The ideal system can remove pressure from the supervisor/administrator by making the development of the instrument and process a collaborative effort with staff and by removing confrontational components. Evaluation can become an experience to look forward to rather than avoided because it is concise and clear and there is no anticipation of adversarial confrontation.

Since adapting to this "new way of doing business" is not easy for some supervisors/administrators, there is an obvious need for the organization to be proactive in the planning and provision of training for these managerial requirements. Providing an early and intensive orientation for supervisors/administrators which outlines the expectations, intentions, and purposes of the system is required. We have had the luxury of involving the same managerial staff for the majority of evaluations and this group was also involved in the development of the system. It became clear, however, that as new supervisors were hired and as we worked with other organizations to implement this system, training was required to help the supervisors/administrators understand the underlying philosophy. In many ways, this constituted a paradigm shift for these individuals.

In every organization there are supervisors and administrators who have an imperious attitude about evaluation and see it primarily as a tool for the elimination of non-performers in the organization. We have no problem with the termination of non-performers (as we have attempted to make clear throughout this text) but that is not the main intent of this system.

Not all managerial staff will be capable of making the shifts required of the ideal system. As a result, there will be pressure upon higher levels of the organization to deal with this issue and to act in a manner that is consistent with the overall philosophy. The ideal system allows this process to occur in the same way with supervisory/administrative conduct as it does with direct service providers.

The same instrument and process can be used to address the non-performing manager.

ORGANIZATIONAL CONSIDERATIONS IN THE IDEAL SYSTEM

We have previously pointed out that the ideal system takes time and considerable investment of human resources to build and maintain. The long-term gains are well worth the pain of assembly, however, and the maintenance is modest if it is handled in a planned and thoughtful way. The ideal system is not built and then allowed to operate without such maintenance because it needs to be adapted to the changes in the service system and the personnel. In fact this is one of the strengths of the ideal system–it can accommodate to changes without a significant alteration of the heart of the model.

This system was developed for a children's mental health setting but we would argue that it can be applied to a wide range of human service systems. The system where it was developed is a diverse one, employing a variety of professional groups including residential child care workers, psychologists, and social workers, to name only a few. The agency serves a broad range of age groups from toddlers to adolescents and their families. There are programs offering acute crisis intervention, school consultation, and preventative services as well.

Within this complex system, the ideal performance evaluation system has been utilized effectively by all staff and administrative personnel. We think that it is easily portable to other human service agencies including family counseling agencies, child protective services, health and hospital systems, educational organizations, residential treatment centers, or almost any system which employs human service providers.

One point worth considering from an organizational perspective is staff retention. Staff who are evaluated by a system which they perceive to be responsive and just are more likely to stay with the organization. One way that staff receive a message about their worth and their importance to the organization is through a responsive evaluation system. To allow them the opportunity to become further empowered through the building and development of the tool and the process can add to their sense of partnership with the organization. This has obvious economic benefits to the organization and will pay for the time and commitment needed to produce the ideal system many times over.

An attractive aspect of the system for the organization is that because the same instrument and process is utilized across the agency, it is possible to compare programs in a consistent manner. The identification of staff development issues and training needs is aided enormously by such congruency. In like manner, the results of evaluation can be used internally for program evaluation purposes. Indeed, we believe there is tremendous research applicability to the ideal system, not only within a single organization but in utilizing it for cross-organizational comparisons.

References

Atkin, R.S. and Conlon, E.J. (1978). Behaviorally anchored rating scales: Some theoretical issues. *Academy of Management Review, 3,* 119-128.

Baker, H.K. and Holmgren, S.R. (1982). Stepping up to supervision: Conducting performance reviews. *Supervisory Management, 27*(4), 20-28.

Bechman, C.W. (1981). Performance appraisal challenges in mental health services. *Journal of Mental Health Administration, 8*(1), 24-26.

Beer, M. (1981). Performance appraisal: Dilemmas and possibilities. *Organizational Dynamics, 9*(3), 24-36.

Bernardin, H.J. and Beatty, R.W. (1984). *Performance appraisal: Assessing human behavior at work.* Boston: Kent Publishing.

Bok, D. (1990). *Universities and the future of America.* Durham, NC: Duke University Press.

Boyer, E.L. (1990). *Scholarship reconsidered: Priorities of the professorate.* Princeton, NJ: The Carnegie Foundation for the Advancement of Teaching.

Brito v. Zia Company, 478 F. 2d. 1200 (1973).

Brumback, G.B. (1988). Some ideas, issues, and predictions about performance management. *Public Personnel Management, 17*(4), 387-402.

Burke, R.J., Wetzel, N., and Weir, T. (1978). Characteristics of effective employee performance review and development interviews: Replication and extension. *Personnel Psychology, 31,* 903-919.

Caroll, S.J. and Schneier, C.E. (1982). *Performance appraisal and review systems.* Glenview, IL: Scott, Foresman.

Cedarblom, D. (1982). The performance appraisal interview: A review, implications, and suggestions. *Academy of Management Review, 7,* 219-227.

Civil Rights Act of 1964, 7, U.S.C. Section 701.

Civil Service Reform Act of 1978, 5, U.S.C. Section 430.

Cronbach, L.J. (1970). *Essentials of psychological testing.* (3rd ed.) New York: Harper and Row.

Cummings, L.L. and Schwab, D.P. (1973). *Performance in organizations: Determinants and appraisal.* Glenview, IL: Scott Foresman.

DeMarco, J.J. and Nigro, L.G. (1983). Using employee attitudes and perceptions to maintain supervisory implementation of CSRA performance appraisal systems. *Public Personnel Management Journal, 12*(1), 43-51.

Dipboye, R.L. and de Pontbriand, R. (1981). Correlates of employee reactions to performance appraisals and appraisal systems. *Journal of Applied Psychology, 66,* 248-251.

Evans, E. and McShane, S.L. (1988). Employee perceptions of performance appraisal fairness in two organizations. *Canadian Journal of Behavioral Science, 20*(2), 177-191.

Ferris, G.R. (1982). The performance evaluation process: Implications of supervisor-subordinate attributional congruency for subordinate work attitudes. *Dissertation Abstracts International, 43,* 862A (University Microfilms No. 82-18, 464).

Flanagan, J.C. (1954). The critical incident technique. *Psychological Bulletin, 51,* 327-358.

Folger, R. and Greenberg, J. (1985). Procedural justice: An interpretive analysis of personnel systems. In K.M. Rowland and G.R. Ferris (Eds.), *Research in personnel and human resource management, Vol. III.* Greenwich, CT: JAI Press. pp. 141-185.

Gilley, J.W. (1990). *The interactive university: A source of American revitalization.* Washington, DC: American Association of State Colleges and Universities.

Greenberg, J. (1986). Determinants of perceived fairness of performance evaluation. *Journal of Applied Psychology, 71,* 340-342.

Harkness, L. and Mulinski, P. (1988). Performance standards for social workers. *Social Work, 33*(4), 339-344.

Jacques, E. (1976). *A general theory of bureaucracy.* New York: Halstead Press.

Kadushin, A. (1968). Games people play in supervision. *Social Work, 13*(3), 23-32.

Kagle, J.D. (1979). Evaluating social work practice. *Social Work,* 24(4), 292-296.

Kane, M.T. (1982). The validity of licensure examinations. *American Psychologist, 37*(8), 911-918.

Landy, F.J., Barnes, J.L., and Murphy, K.R. (1978). Correlates of perceived fairness and accuracy of performance evaluation. *Journal of Applied Psychology, 63,* 751-754.

Landy, F.J. and Farr, J.L. (1983). *The measurement of work performance: Methods, theory, and applications.* New York: Academic Press.

Latham, G.P. and Wexley, K.N. (1981). *Increasing productivity through performance appraisal.* Reading, MA: Addison-Wesley.

Levine, H.Z. (1986). Performance appraisal at work. *Personnel, 63*(6), 63-71.

Levinson, H. (1979). Management of what performance? *Harvard Business Review: On human relations.* New York: Harper and Row.

Lombardi, D.N. (1988). *Handbook of personnel selection and performance evaluation in health care.* San Francisco: Jossey-Bass.

MacIntosh, J. (1988). Staff appraisal. *Physiotherapy, 74*(2), 95-97.

Marsh, J. C. and Weick, A. (1992). Point/Counterpoint: Should publication productivity be the primary criterion for tenure decisions? *Journal of Social Work Education, 28*(2), 132-140.

McGregor, D. (1972). An uneasy look at performance appraisal. *Harvard Business Review, 50*(5), 133-138.

Millar, K., Matheson, W., and Van Dyk, C. (1989). *Performance appraisal of staff in a child and youth service agency.* Paper presented at the Annual Conference of The National Association of Social Workers, San Francisco, CA, October 1989, (unpublished).

Millar, K. (1988). *The development and field test of behaviorally anchored rating scales for evaluating performance of professional social workers.* Unpublished doctoral dissertation, University of Texas at Arlington, Arlington, TX.

Millar, K. (1990). Performance appraisal of professional social workers. *Administration in Social Work, 14*(1), 65-85.

Mohrman, Jr., A.M., Resnick-West, S.M., and Lawler III, E.E. (1989). *Designing performance appraisal systems*. San Francisco: Jossey-Bass.

Nemeroff, W.F. and Wexley, K.N. (1979). An exploration of the relationships between performance feedback interview characteristics and interview outcomes as perceived by managers and subordinates. *Journal of Occupational Psychology, 52*(1), 25-34.

Patten, T. (1976). Linking financial rewards to employee performance: The roles of O.D. and M.B.O. *Human Resource Management, 15*(Winter), 2-17.

Patz, A. (1975). Performance appraisal: Useful but still resisted. *Harvard Business Review, 53*(3), 74-80.

Peters, T. (1985). *The no-win world of performance appraisal*. Palo Alto, CA: The Tom Peters Group.

Pottinger, P.S. and Goldsmith, N. (1979). *Defining and measuring competencies: New directions for experimental learning*. San Francisco: Jossey-Bass.

Rasmussen, J. (1988). Occupational therapy staff evaluation: A personnel and program management system. In *The occupational therapy manager's handbook*. New York: The Haworth Press. pp. 23-31.

Rendero, T. (1980). Performance appraisal practices. *Personnel, 57*(6), 4-12.

Rivas, R.F. (1984). Perspectives on dismissal as a management prerogative in social service organizations. *Administration in Social Work, 8*, (4), 77-92.

Rock, M. (1972). *Handbook of wage and salary administration*. New York: McGraw-Hill.

Sashkin, M. (1981). Appraising appraisal: Ten lessons from research to practice. *Organizational Dynamics, 9*(3), 24-36.

Schwab, D.P., Heneman III, H.G., and DeCotiis, T. (1975). Behaviorally anchored rating scales: A review of the literature. *Personnel Psychology, 28*, 549-562.

Smith, P.C. (1976). Behaviors, results, and organizational effectiveness: The problem of criteria. In M.D. Dunnette (Ed.), *Handbook of industrial and organizational psychology*. Chicago: Rand McNally. pp. 745-775.

Smith, P.C. and Kendall, L.F. (1963). Retranslation of expectations: An approach to the construction of unambiguous anchors for rating scales. *Journal of Applied Psychology, 47,* 149-155.

Spano, R.M. (1981). Performance appraisal in a hospital social service department. *Social Work in Health Care, 7*(2), 13-37.

Thorndike, R. and Hagen, E. (1977). *Measurement and evaluation in psychology and education* (4th ed.). New York: John Wiley & Sons.

Timmreck, T.C. (1989). Performance appraisal systems in rural western hospitals. *Health Care Management Review, 14*(2), 31-43.

Wade v. Mississippi Cooperative Extension Service, 372 F. Supp. 126 (1974).

Wexley, K.N., Singh, J.P., and Yukl, G.A. (1973). Subordinate personality as a moderator of the effects of participation in three types of appraisal interviews. *Journal of Applied Psychology, 58,* 54-59.

Wexley, K.N. and Yukl, G.A. (1977). *Organizational behavior and personnel psychology.* Homewood, IL: Irwin.

Wiehe, V. (1980). Current practices in performance appraisal. *Administration in Social Work, 4*(3), 1-11.

Index

Abramson, Sally (case study), 17-19
Administration. *See* Management
    and performance evaluation;
    Organizations and
    performance evaluation;
    Supervisors
Adolescent care knowledge, 82
Agencies. *See* Organizations and
    performance evaluation
"Agree to disagree"
    employees' view of, 124-125
    in performance evaluation,
        34-35,47-48,57
    supervisors' view of, 127
À LA CARTE criteria
    agency changes and, 49
    in behaviorally anchored rating
        scales (BARS), 42
    case study, 14,17-18
    constructing, 45-46,124
    vs. CORE criteria, 26-27
    in ideal performance evaluation,
        25-27
    identification by staff, 44-45
    new employees, 114-115
    for new positions, 48-49
    program managers, 117-118
    sample instrument, 52-53,54
        agency advocacy and service
            integration, 90-91
        child and adolescent care, 82
        client relationships, 74-75
        communication skills, 81
        coordination of services, 92-93
        external consultative service
            provision, 79-80
        fiscal planning and
            management, 88-89

À LA CARTE criteria, sample
    instrument *(continued)*
        human resources management,
            84-85
        intervention plan
            implementation, 78
        intervention plan selection, 77
        office practice, 94
        problem identification and
            assessment, 76
        program planning, 86-87
        score sheet, 96-97
        teamwork, 83
        understanding of, 55-56
    senior employees, 116-117
Applicability of performance
    evaluation, 25-26
Audiotapes in performance tests, 8

Baker, H.K., 30
Barnes, J.L., 31
BARS. *See* Behaviorally anchored
    rating scales
Bechman, C.W., 40
Behavioral statements, 39-40
Behaviorally anchored rating scales
    (BARS), 8-9. *See also*
    Benchmarks
    case study, 17-19
    characteristics, 41-43
    construction with staff
        participation, 43-46
    performance evaluation process,
        46-50
    sample instrument, 54-55,95-98

Benchmarks
  administrative requirements and
      professional growth, 24-25
  agency requirements, 27-28
  case study, 18
  constructing, 43
  growth and loss of function, 36
  sample instrument, 55
  scores below, 104
  in synoptic method, 109
Biases
  in critical incident techniques, 8
  in trait-based rating scales, 7
Bok, D., ix
Boyer, E.L., ix
Brito v. Zia Company, 5
Brumback, G.B., 24
Budget/fiscal planning and
      management, 88-89

Canada's Bill of Rights, 5
Case studies
  Abramson, Sally, 17-19
  Webster, Ian, 13-17
Cedarblom, D., 24
Child care knowledge, 82
Civil Rights Act, 5
Client relationships, 74-75
Client services, 90-93
Clinical providers, 124
Clinical team review, 120-122
Colleague relationships, 59,82
Communication. *See* Dialogue
Communication skills, 81
Community resources, 66
Compensation and performance
      evaluation
  case study, 15
  disassociating, 28-29,44
Consultation, use of, 71
Consultative service, 79-80
CORE criteria
  agency changes and, 49
  vs. À LA CARTE criteria, 25-27

CORE criteria *(continued)*
  in behaviorally anchored rating
      scales (BARS), 42
  constructing, 45-46
  identification by staff, 44-45
  new employees, 114-115
  program managers, 117-118
  reflection of organizational
      concerns, 125
  sample instrument, 52,54
    awareness of organization
        policies, 62-63
    colleague relationships, 59
    consultation and supervision
        use, 71
    knowledge of community
        resources, 66
    knowledge of target population,
        61
    professional development,
        69,72-73
    public relations, 64-65
    relationships with other
        organizations, 60
    score sheet, 95-96
    time management, 70
    understanding of, 55-56
    values and ethics, 67-68
  senior employees, 116-117
Critical incident techniques, 8
Criticism in performance evaluation,
    23
Cummings, L.L., 2

DeCotiis, T., 37
DeMarco, J.J., 37
de Pontbriand, R., 37
Dialogue
  clinical team review, 122
  employees' view of, 124-125
  in performance evaluation,
      34-35,47-48,57
  with problematic employee, 120
  scores below benchmark, 104
  sharing scores, 103-104

Dimensions. *See* À LA CARTE criteria; CORE criteria
Dipboye, R.L., 37
Discrimination laws, 5
Discussion. *See* Dialogue

Education. *See* Professional growth and development
Employee retention, 32,129-130
Employees, new, 100-101,113-115
Employees and performance evaluation
  attitudes toward organization, 10
  behaviorally anchored rating scales (BARS), 43-46
  changes in personal development, 35-36
  colleague relationships, 59
  considerations in, 123-126
  constructing, 17,29-31
  fairness of, 37
  independent evaluation, 33-34
  meeting needs in, 9-10
  meeting with supervisors, 47-48
  motivation and, 5
  organization's attitude toward, 23-24
  orientation and performance evaluation, 48-49
  orientation phase, 100-101
  personalized performance evaluation, 37-38
  role in goal setting, 105
  single performance evaluation system, 38-39
  synoptic and focused performance
    new employees, 113-115
    problematic employee, 118-120
    program manager, 117-118
    senior employee, 115-117
  systemic method, 120-122
  teamwork, 83
  training, 5
  trait-based rating scales, 25

Equal Employment Opportunity Commission, 5
Ethics, 67-68
Evans, E., 30,37

Face-to-face meeting, 47-48,103
  focused method, 110-111
  scores below benchmark, 104
  synoptic method, 108-109
  time in process, 102
Fairness of performance evaluation, 37
Farr, J.L., 40
Fiscal/budget planning and management, 88-89
Flanagan, J.C., 41-42
Focused method
  clinical team review, 121-122
  new employee, 113-115
  problematic employee, 118-120
  program manager, 117-118
  senior employee, 115-117
  use of, 110-111
Folger, R., 37
Forced distribution evaluation system, 7
Frequency of performance evaluation, 101
Future component, 32-33,38. *See also* Goal setting

Generic criteria. *See* CORE criteria
Gilley, J.W., ix
Goal setting, 105
  case study, 16
  future component, 32-33,38
  in performance evaluation, 38
  time in process, 101-102
  timing of, 57-58
Goldsmith, N., 30
Greenberg, J., 37

"Halo effect," 7,8
Heneman, H.G., III, 37

Hierarchical model, 125,127-128
Holmgren, S.R., 30
Human resources management,
    84-85

Independent component, 47,102
Interactive University, ix
Internal transfers, 100
Intervention plan
    implementation and evaluation, 78
    selection, 77

Jacques, E., 23
Job dimensions. *See* À LA CARTE
    criteria; CORE criteria
Job-specific criteria. *See* À LA
    CARTE criteria
Joint assessment, 34

Kane, M.T., 30
Kendall, L.F., 41-42

Landy, F.J., 31, 40
Language of performance evaluation
    case study, 14,17
    characteristics, 29
    in constructing, 45
    dimensions, 56
Latham, G.P., 4,5
Legal considerations of performance
    evaluation, 2,4
    behavioral content, 31
    discrimination, 5
    U.S. Civil Service Reform Act of
        1978, 5-6
Levinson, H., 32
Lombardi, D.N., 22,25,28,31

MacIntosh, J., 33
Management and performance
    evaluation. *See also*
    Supervisors

Management and performance
    evaluation *(continued)*
    development of, 17,30
    future component, 32-33
    responsibility for, 4
    use of systemic method, 112-113
Management functions
    agency advocacy and service
        integration, 90-91
    fiscal/budget planning, 88-89
    human resources, 84-85
    program planning, development
        and evaluation, 86-87
Matheson, W., 9
McGregor, D., 2,23,28
McShane, S.L., 30,37
Millar, K., 9
Murphy, K.R., 31

Negativism in performance
    evaluation, 23
Nigro, L.G., 37
1964 Civil Rights Act, 5
Non-punitive performance
    evaluation systems, 22-24,45
Numerical components, 39-40

Office practice skills, 94
Organization of time and work, 70
Organizations and performance
    evaluation
    benchmarks, 24,27-28,43
    changes in, 39,49
    considerations, 129-130
    reflection of philosophy in,
        23-24,125
    sample instrument
        agency advocacy and service
            integration, 90-91
        awareness of policies and
            services, 62-63
        consultation and supervision
            use, 71
        knowledge of target population,
            61

Organizations and performance
evaluation, sample instrument
(continued)
  public relations, 64-65
  relationships with other
    organizations, 60
  staff development opportunities,
    72-73
  systemic method, 111-113
  training of supervisors/
    administrators, 128
Orientation phase,
    48-49,100-101,102

Paired comparison evaluation
    system, 7
Pay and performance evaluation
  case study, 15
  disassociating, 28-29,44
Performance evaluation
  applicability to position, 14,17
  behaviorally anchored rating
    scales (BARS), 41-50
    characteristics, 41-43
    construction, 43-46
    evaluation process, 46-50
  case studies
    Abramson, Sally, 17-19
    Webster, Ian, 13-17
  characteristics of ideal, 21-40
    adaptability with agency
      change, 39
    administrative requirements and
      professional growth, 24-25
    applicability for all staff, 38-39
    availability, 36-37
    benchmark of agency
      expectation, 27-28
    fairness, 37
    fast and efficient, 33
    future-oriented, 32-33
    goal orientation, 38
    growth and loss of function,
      35-36
    high content validity, 37

Performance evaluation,
  characteristics of ideal *(continued)*
    independent component, 33-34
    job-specific and generic criteria,
      25-27
    language, 29
    non-adversarial, 34-35
    pay, 28-29
    personalized experience, 37-38
    positive and non-punitive, 22-24
    real events, 30-31
    semantic and numerical
      components, 39-40
    staff participation, 29-30
    time-framed and repetitive,
      31-32
    user's guide, 32
  difficulties of, 3-4
  employee considerations, 123-126
  examining score profiles, 107-122
    focused method, 110-111
    new employee, 113-115
    problematic employee, 118-120
    program manager, 117-118
    senior employee, 115-117
    synoptic method, 108-109
    systemic method,
      111-113,120-122
  focus of, 9-10
  goals of, 5-6
  implementing, 99-106
    dialogue, 103-104
    face-to-face meeting, 103
    goal setting, 105
    orientation phase, 100-101
    review process, 105-106
    scores below benchmark, 104
    scoring, 102-103
    time frames, 101-102
  importance of, 4
  mechanisms, 6-9
    behaviorally anchored rating
      scales (BARS), 8-9

Performance evaluation, mechanisms
        (continued)
    critical incident techniques, 8
    performance tests, 8
    ranking, paired comparison, and
        forced distribution systems, 7
    trait-based rating scales, 6-7
    organizational considerations,
        129-130
    results of, 1-2
    review of, 105-106,113
    sample instrument, 51-98
        À LA CARTE dimensions,
            52-53,74-94
        CORE dimensions, 52,59-73
        dimensions, 55-56
        evaluation process, 56-57
        goal setting, 57-58
        language, 56
        scale, 54-55
        SCORE SHEET, 95-98
        time boundaries, 56
    supervisor/administrative
        considerations, 126-129
    supervisors' view of, 2-3
Performance tests, 8
Peters, T., 23
Plateau of performance, 35
Positive performance evaluation
        systems, 22-24,45
Pottinger, P.S., 30
Practicality of performance
        evaluation system, 21
Problem identification and
        assessment, 76
Professional growth and
        development
    À LA CARTE criteria, 24-28
    benchmarks, 43
    changes in, 35-36
    future component of performance
        evaluation, 33
    of managers in ideal performance
        evaluation, 128
    performance evaluation in, 5

Professional growth and
        development *(continued)*
    responsibility for, 69,72-73
Professional values and ethics, 67-68
Program managers, 117-118
Program planning, 86-87
Public relations, 64-65

Quality control of performance
        evaluation system,
        105-106,113

Ranking evaluation system, 7
Reliability of performance
        evaluation system, 21
Repetition of performance
        evaluation, 31-32
Review of performance evaluation
        system, 105-106,113
Rivas, R.F., 3

Sashkin, M., 27-28,33
Scale, sample instrument, 54-55
Schools of social work, ix
Schwab, D.P., 2,37
Scientific approach, x
Score sheet, sample, 95-98
Scoring profiles, 102-104
    synoptic and focused method,
        108-111
        new employee, 113-115
        problematic employee, 118-120
        program manager, 117-118
        senior employee, 115-117
    systemic method,
        111-113,120-122
Self-development
    À LA CARTE criteria, 24-28
    benchmarks, 43
    measuring in performance
        evaluation, 35-36
Semantic components, 39-40,43
Smith, P.C., 41-42

South Cochrane Child and Youth
  Service, x
Spano, R.M., 30,38
Staff. *See* Employees
Supervisors. *See also* Management
    and performance evaluation
  considerations in performance
    evaluation system, 126-129
  dealing with scores below
    benchmark, 104
  in focused method, 110-111,115
  in goal setting, 105
  human resources management,
    84-85
  meeting with employees, 47-48
  orientation phase of performance
    evaluation system, 101
  performance evaluation, 117-118
  problematic employees, 119
  program planning, development
    and evaluation, 86-87
  relationship to employees, 125
  in synoptic method, 108-109,115
  use of, 71
  view of performance evaluation,
    2-3
Synoptic method
  clinical team review, 121-122
  new employee, 113-115
  program manager, 117-118
  senior employee, 115-117
  use of, 108-109
Systemic method, 111-113
  clinical team review, 120-122

Target population
  knowledge of, 61
  knowledge of services and policies
    toward, 62-63

Teamwork, 83
Time-frame of performance
    evaluation, 31-32,33,56,
    101-102
Time management, 70
Timmreck, T.C., 34
Traditional trait-based rating scales.
    See Trait-based rating scales
Training. *See* Professional growth
    and development
Trait-based rating scales, 6-7,25
  case study, 14-15
Transferred employees, 100

University
  interactive, ix
  role in the community, ix
U.S. Civil Service Reform Act of
    1978, 5-6
User's guide, 32,49

Validity of performance evaluation
    system, 21,37
Values, 67-68
Van Dyk, C., 9
Video tapes in performance tests, 8

*Wade v. Mississippi Cooperative
    Extension Service*, 5
Webster, Ian (case study), 13-17
Weick, Ann, x
Wexley, K.N., 4,5,33,38
Wording. *See* Language of
    performance evaluation

Yukl, G.A., 33,38